Grief and AIDS

To my Father

Ceymon Samuel

Grief and AIDS

Edited by

Lorraine Sherr

Royal Free Hospital School of Medicine, London, UK

JOHN WILEY & SONS

Chichester · New York · Brisbane · Toronto · Singapore

Other Wiley Editorial Offices

John Wiley & Sons, Inc., 605 Third Avenue,
New York, NY 10158-0012, USA

Jacaranda Wiley Ltd, 33 Park Road, Milton,
Queensland 4064, Australia

John Wiley & Sons (Canada) Ltd, 22 Worcester Road,
Rexdale, Ontario M9W 1L1, Canada

John Wiley & Sons (SEA) Pte Ltd, 37 Jalan Pemimpin #05-04,
Block B, Union Industrial Building, Singapore 2057

Library of Congress Cataloging-in-Publication Data
Grief and AIDS / edited by Lorraine Sherr.
    p. cm.
  Includes bibliographical references and index.
  ISBN 0-471-95346-6 (paper)
    1. AIDS (Disease)—Psychological aspects. 2. Grief.
  3. Bereavement. I. Sherr, Lorraine.
  RC607.A26G776 1995
  362.1'969792'0019—dc20   94–38635
                                                    CIP

British Library Cataloguing in Publication Data
A catalogue record for this book is available from the British Library

ISBN 0-471-95346-6 (paper)

Typeset in 10/12pt Palatino by Dobbie Typesetting Limited, Tavistock, Devon
Printed and bound in Great Britain by Bookcraft (Bath) Ltd
This book is printed on acid-free paper responsibly manufactured from sustainable
forestation, for which at least two trees are planted for each one used for paper production.

Contents

About the Editor

Lorraine Sherr........... Royal Free Hospital School of Medicine, University of London, Department of Public Health, Rowland Hill Street, London NW3 2PF, UK

Lorraine Sherr is a Senior Lecturer and Head of Health Psychology at the Royal Free Hospital School of Medicine (London University). She co-edits the International Journal *AIDS Care* and is the founding editor of *Psychology Health and Medicine*. She has published numerous books on AIDS and HIV infection and also on grief-related issues such as *HIV Infection in Mothers and Babies* (Blackwell 1991); *AIDS In the Heterosexual Population* (Harwood 1993); and *Death, Dying and Bereavement* (Blackwell 1989).

Dr Sherr was awarded a Churchill Fellowship to examine AIDS and HIV infection in Africa and has carried out a number of research projects. She has also been involved in clinical care at St Mary's Hospital from the start of the epidemic. She is chair of the British Psychological Society Special Interest Group in AIDS and also one of the organizers of the International AIDS Impact meetings.

Contributors

Lydia Bennett .... Department of Behaviour and Social Sciences, Building M02, University of Sydney, NSW 2006, Australia

J Catalan .... Department of Psychiatry, Chelsea and Westminster Hospital, 369 Fulham Road, London SW10 9NH, UK

L Dean .... School of Public Health, Sociomedical Sciences, AIDS Research Unit, Columbia University in the City of New York, New York 10027, USA

Calliope C. S. Farsides.... University of Keele, Keele, Staffordshire ST5 5BG, UK

Ellen Kajura .... MRC, UVRI, PO Box 49, Entebbe, Uganda

C Mead .... Faculteit der Sociale Wetenschappen, Vakgroep Klinische Gezondheids en Persoonlijkheid Psychologies, Rijksuniversiteit, Wassenaarseweg 52, Leiden, The Netherlands

K Pugh .... Department of Psychiatry, The Maudsley Hospital, Denmark Hill, London SE5 8AF, UK

M Reidy............... Faculté des Sciences Infirmières, University of Montreal CP 6128, Succursale Centre Ville, Montreal, Quebec, Canada

A Richardson .... City Hospital, 51 Greenbank Drive, Edinburgh EH10 5SB, UK

Brigitte Richmond........ University of New South Wales, Sydney, Australia

Michael W. Ross......... University of Texas at Houston, Center for Health Education Research and Development, School of Public Health, PO Box 20186, Houston, Texas 77225, USA

Janet Seeley .... MRC, UVRI, PO Box 49, Entebbe, Uganda

M. F. van den Boom ..... Blood Transfusion Council of the Netherlands Red Cross, Plesmanlaan 125, NL-1066 CX, The Netherlands

Hessel W. A. Willemsen .. Rijksuniversiteit, Wassenaarseweg 52, Leiden, The Netherlands

Preface

The burden of grief is the silent backdrop that looms behind the high profile AIDS and HIV epidemic. As the relentless disease process lumbers on it leaves a catalogue of loss and grief in its wake. Although humanity has faced grief in different forms throughout time, this new international loss will challenge the caring facilities of all. It will prove to be the great leveller from the artistic communities in the USA to the drug users on the lower East Side, Scotland, Europe and Asia; the refugees, the African truck drivers; the Thai street-workers; the infants, the teenagers, the men, the women, and the elderly. All, and more, will face elements of AIDS-associated grief and need to forge life in its presence.

This text is an attempt to explore many of the notions of grief and AIDS. The mantle spreads widely. There are different perspectives – those who are bereaved as they lose a parent, a child, a partner, a lover, or a patient. Grief and loss may be an internal experience as the natural history of HIV disease hurtles individuals from one loss to another. The grief may ramify broadly as it touches multiple members of families and networks leaving a marred path in its wake. Psychological and social functioning may be dramatically affected by the extent and level of grief any individual, group, or community is contending with.

Yet there have been some enormously enriching programmes which have rallied to the call. There has been an awareness of the specific and general needs, and a variety of innovative attempts to meet these. There are those who argue that HIV and AIDS is very special, unique, and different. On the other hand there are those who turn to existing bodies of learning, current programmes of help, and try to adapt them and glean from their teachings in order to respond to HIV and AIDS. A balanced approach, gleaning from both, must surely point to the future.

No-one knows what tomorrow holds. The passage of time increases the load which serves to stretch resources to breaking point and results in a weary and saturated set of individuals and organizations who are struggling to cope. At the core is the fact that many of the bereaved are themselves HIV positive – facing their own personal losses and living in a world where their loved ones may have been snatched away. Such a multiple burden has little precedent, and workers are unsure how to react and what to anticipate. The only lessons are to avoid denial.

This book is an attempt to examine a wide range of grief-related issues as it affects people with HIV infection and AIDS. It provides a psychological focus which concentrates on the impact of the individuals and examines a number of interventions at the counselling or systems level to address or ameliorate grief. Contributions are collated from workers all over the world – Australia, Africa, Europe, Canada and the USA. The first chapter (Sherr) is an overview of counselling and bereavement, which sets out to explore psychological concepts of grief and to evaluate interventions. It examines a number of notions, specifically psychological concepts in grief, duration and stages of grieving and whether these notions are helpful. Other elements include anticipatory grief, social support and numerous practical issues. Dean (Chapter 2) provides an overview of the impact of death and dying on the gay community in New York as grief unfolds over time. Grief and loss takes many forms and Pugh (Chapter 3) examines issues associated with suicide and AIDS. Suicide is a difficult notion to quantify and understand, yet the burden of suicidal thoughts and acts may have a specific impact both on those infected with HIV and on those who survive or are bereaved by an HIV-related suicide. Catalan (Chapter 4) examines the body of knowledge on psychiatric sequelae of bereavement with specific application to HIV infection and AIDS. He provides an overview of factors associated with various types of grief expression, especially disorders where psychiatric management and intervention are required. Seeley and Kajura (Chapter 5) explore the meaning of grief and death at the community level, taking into consideration some of the large-scale losses in African communities. This chapter eloquently describes some of the social burden and explores elements of rites, burial and compounding factors such as economic hardship and loneliness. They examine the place of counselling and support services. Bennett (Chapter 6) gives an overview of knowledge and experience of grief as it affects staff and carers. She explores some of the notions associated with disenfranchised grief and how stigma and discrimination ramify onto staff. She explores the notion of burnout and how it may potentially affect HIV and AIDS carers, especially given the number of deaths they are exposed to, the feelings of responsibility they foster, the current lack of a cure and the high level of identification with people living with AIDS. This chapter also reminds workers of the positive aspects of caring for people with AIDS and how a balanced approach can ensure a productive relationship. Farsides (Chapter 7) pursues some of the ethical issues surrounding the need to allow someone to die. She contrasts the medical and ethical models of care and explores the notions of quality versus quantity of life. The notions are not straightforward and there are many challenges embodied in the options of choice, proxy decision-making, means and acts which drive the practicalities of palliative care. Mead and Willemsen (Chapter 8) give a psychodynamic perspective of AIDS-related loss and raise notions of mortality and crisis.

End-of-life issues are challenging in the day-to-day care of people with HIV infection and AIDS. Richardson (Chapter 9) explores the use of living wills for this group and how the process facilitates control, choice and dialogue. A number of case vignettes are used to explore notions of treatment refusal, decision making, conflicting opinions, resuscitation orders, mental impairment and control. Van den Boom (Chapter 10) explores the grief issues associated with the loss of a parent. This chapter examines both the short- and long-term effects of parental death, and attempts to understand determinants of psychopathology. An understanding of intervention programmes, guidance and support groups is given to help understand the family – whether infected, uninfected or affected.

Richmond and Ross (Chapter 11) set out some of the issues associated with the death of a partner. Much of their data is drawn from interview studies which explore common themes, positive experiences with bereavement and examine how bereavement affects survivors' lives and how survivors change their own lives after bereavement with concerns about their own future and often in the face of both personal HIV infection and bereavement overload. Finally, Reidy (Chapter 12) examines the wide-reaching implications of the death of a child.

This text is by no means comprehensive. It attempts to draw on a wide body of literature and front-line experience to assist those in contemplating care and death. It aims to allow the reader to become aware of the many facets of grief, on the assumption that insight and understanding may lighten the load.

Acknowledgements

A book on Grief and AIDS may be a time to acknowledge many people who by their courage, tenacity, inspiration or example have roused the sleeping multitude to sit up and examine the very essence of life. I look around me and need to thank many of these. John Campbell has led by example. Sue Newman showed me what fighting spirit was all about. I am surrounded by colleagues who provide daily vitality and who teach me that lateral thinking may win through. Sue Quinn, Lindsay Neil, Catherine Peckham, Di Melvin and Lydia Bennett are just a few who make the word 'colleague' an asset. Janis Hodges and Elaine Harris create the efficient backbone without which functioning would simply cease.

I would also like to acknowledge the HEA, whose grant on *Suicide and AIDS* served to inform some of my work, as well as the European Community, which provided a trigger for much of the work by allowing the exchange of ideas and information on their Biomed I project on AIDS and Ethics.

As always the patience and competition for the computer was shared by Ari, Ilan, Yonatan and Liora. Without Avrom all this would never be possible.

CHAPTER 1

The Experience of Grief – Psychological Aspects of Grief in AIDS and HIV infection

Lorraine Sherr

*Royal Free Hospital School of Medicine,
London, UK*

Much has emerged in the wake of the AIDS pandemic, but the trail of grief for the individual, the family and the community has been so widespread and profound that it may mar the psyche of generations to come.

There is nothing new about grief, and the existing body of learning must be adapted to accommodate and adjust for those touched by AIDS and HIV infection. What is new is the nature of this disease, the groups it affects, the societal reaction to it, and the compound nature of the burden it brings. This chapter sets out to examine some death and bereavement reactions and options, together with responses and counselling guidance. There are few magic formulas and in the end death is often, inevitably, a personal event. Yet there is much around the process that can be helped, supported or simply confronted, where knowledge can replace ignorance and action can substitute denial.

The mantle of grief extends in a variety of ways. Initially there is the grief affecting the individual who is diagnosed with HIV infection, proceeds to AIDS or faces terminal illness. Simultaneous to this process is the grief felt by those around them – their partners, their loved ones, their family, their community and their carers. Grief is not a single concept but meanders in many forms through the course of this disease. This very fact means that the effects of grief are cumulative and add disproportionately to the load.

Grief and AIDS. Edited by L. Sherr.
©1995 John Wiley & Sons Ltd.

PSYCHOLOGICAL CONCEPTS IN GRIEF

The complexity of grief has been the subject of wide-ranging theoretical formulation, despite the fact that feelings of sadness and depression on losing someone or something loved are 'self evident' (Stroebe, Stroebe and Hansson 1993).

Grief comprises the emotional reactions focused on or surrounding the longing for someone or something that is no longer there. Its presence is most often studied in terms of death, but there are many other situations in which dramatic permanent absence is countenanced.

The theories, as they stand, are rather piecemeal. Stroebe and Stroebe (1993) describe strands of theory emanating from:

- A depression model base
- A stress theory base
- An emotion model
- A disease-based medical model

Such Sherrtheories are limited in terms of explanations unless they can provide some guided intervention pathways. Parkes (1993) focuses on adaptation to grief situations and emphasizes the role of professionals and carers in facilitating change during the experience of grieving.

Stages of Grieving

The literature is peppered with theories that outline stages and phases in the grieving process. Although these are helpful in describing the emotions and experiences of a number of individuals, they need to be used with caution. They can never incorporate the nuances of every individual experience. The mere provision of stages or phases is enticing as a means to simplify and compartmentalize what in essence is a diverse and complex series of enormously powerful emotions. The stages are useful in describing and defining the range and extent of the emotional experiences, but are limited when invoked literally without the flexibility to adjust and accommodate individual variation. Furthermore, this form of theory imposes a somewhat passive reaction on the dying. With AIDS the diagnosis usually affects younger people who may be ill-prepared for death and may have spent little time contemplating life issues, let alone their own mortality. There may be many active processes that they invoke to accommodate the notion of mortality and adjust their life-styles on hearing of their diagnosis. Some adjustments may be adaptive and assist the individual with coping. Some may reduce pain or trauma and may facilitate the quality of remaining life. Other individuals may not undergo such adaptation for reasons which are unclear, as is the effect.

An innovative progression can be seen in the work of Worden (1991) who reinterprets some of the stage-bound ideas into a series of tasks. This formulation allows for an active evaluation of grieving, and also allows for access for the individual and helpers to facilitate such tasks, either by providing input or by expanding the skill repertoire of the individual who is suddenly faced with a strange and demanding series of events.

Duration

Most studies examining grief duration look at the problem in a linear rather than a cumulative way. They presume a single, sudden loss and in these circumstances attempt to quantify duration range over a variety of emotional responses. For example, two studies of widows found considerable emotional expression after a year (Parkes 1971; Bornstein et al 1973). More insightful accounts (Goin, Burgoyne and Goin 1979; Schuchter and Zisook 1993) examine the lifelong aspects of grief. It thus seems helpful to suggest that grief is for ever – once a loss has been sustained its permanence has to be integrated into the daily psyche of the affected individual.

Time limits and duration factors are more useful when examining intensity of reaction, level of interference with daily living and the extent to which grief impedes, hinders and numbs functioning in the outside world.

Anticipatory Grief

There is a notion that grief is not simply reactive to a loss, but may be triggered as a process in anticipation of a loss. This notion may have interesting implications for adaptation and preparation and may also explain a variety of reactions after a loss. Anticipatory grieving, for example, has been shown to trigger a diverse range of emotions in those involved in grieving and in the caring staff. Natterson and Knudson (1960) noted that when the family of a dying individual came to acceptance prior to the actual death, staff exhibited simultaneous anger and experienced stress. HIV infection is unique in its extensive period of infection. Thus there would, theoretically, be time for an anticipatory grieving process to be set in motion. Literature on sudden death has examined the benefits (if any) of preparation. These may shed light on the notion of anticipatory grief. However, they may be difficult to interpret or generalize because wide-ranging methodological problems make generalizations very difficult. Some studies have noted a negative effect of unexpected loss (Stroebe and Stroebe 1987; Sanders 1983), while other studies have failed to confirm this (Beckenridge et al 1986). These findings may have particular relevance given that many people with AIDS only find out about their HIV status on first diagnosis of an opportunistic infection. This may be particularly true for groups who do not consider themselves at special risk.

Social Support

Social support is a concept that is often raised in the debate on bereavement. It is seen as a factor to facilitate bereavement recovery and aid adjustment to dying. However, it is a concept that is often poorly understood, measured or operationalized. Social support may refer to a variety of supportive elements (House 1981). It may serve multiple functions (Rook 1987) such as the provision of companionship as a buffer against loneliness, as well as promoting social exchange and practical help. It is unclear whether 'social support' is a surrogate marker for personality variables. It may well be that the kind of person who can muster, sustain and utilize social support, may be well disposed to dealing with bereavement for other reasons.

Most workers make presumptions about the presence of beneficial social support. However, there may well be a negative impact on adjustment for mistargeted or unhelpful social support. The components cannot be isolated from their source. Thoits (1985) points out that similar advice may be interpreted as either helpful or overjudgemental dependent on source. Social support should not be seen as a passive commodity that can be administered like a linctus. It is probably a complex phenomenon, which (as stated above) may well reflect personality or circumstantial factors for the supported individual as well. Furthermore, it is clear that it is not a one-way notion of availability. Parkes and Weiss (1983) clarified that the availability of social support needed to be considered in terms of utilization. Indeed, some interesting work (Wethington and Kesler 1986) has shown that support does not even have to be present to have beneficial effects. The key factor for the needy individual was the perception of its availability rather than the level of received support.

Thus it seems that social support is not a simplistic notion. There may be a dynamic aspect to such support, where the needs of the bereaved have to be fine-tuned to the resources of the support if it is to be of use. If there were a clearer understanding of the nature and mechanisms of social support and its positive effect on bereavement adjustment, interventions and training could be more finely tuned. For example, Schilling (1987) noted that there was a fine balance between appropriate support and obstacles to the process of self-reliance.

LOSS AND HIV INFECTION

The course of HIV disease is marked by a catalogue of losses (Green and Sherr 1989). The first point of HIV identification can be traumatic. In an ideal situation HIV is identified by test results following comprehensive counselling and preparation (Miller 1990). Such counselling is aimed to prepare an individual for possible bad news and to set coping strategies into motion in anticipation (Sherr and George 1989). In reality the process may not be effective, the reaction may challenge the coping mechanisms set in place to a greater degree than anticipated and, sadly, often such counselling is simply not present (McCann & Wadsworth 1991; Sherr et al 1993). Cognitive preparation can occur in the absence of counselling and some individuals face the news of HIV positivity with accurate anticipation.

A diagnosis of HIV may result in sudden and dramatic grief over a variety of losses, which are discussed below.

Health

An individual may have to face sudden and unexpected periods of ill health while previously taking good health for granted. This can impose a host of limitations on their everyday life, exacerbated by the constant need to attend for medical check-ups and perhaps take prophylactic medication, all of which serve as a stark reminder of potential ill health.

Relationships

HIV infection can dramatically affect people's relationships as well as the ease with which new relationships may be fostered. However, it is found that individuals often report relationship enhancement in the presence of such challenges.

Sex

As HIV is sexually transmitted, infection with the virus may lead to an unwelcome examination of sexual behaviour and curtailment of previously enjoyed behaviour, and may mark periods of abstinence, psychosexual hurdles and problems. This comes at the very time when the expression of close, warm, loving intimacy may be especially desired.

Future

A diagnosis of HIV serves as an abrupt interruption to an individual's notion of an endless future. This can trigger extensive grief responses and may herald a need to question meaning and attainment and to reappraise direction.

Certainty

Much human endeavour is founded on some degree of certainty, however weakly based this may be. A diagnosis of a dramatic infection such as HIV may call such certainty into question. If this is challenged, much mental anguish, pain and suffering can be experienced in the presence of fears of the unknown and the unanticipated.

Life

HIV infection and AIDS challenge life itself, as well as the investment, plans and meanings that an individual apportions to their life.

Job

Employment is often dramatically affected by HIV infection. On the one extreme, societal prejudice and ignorance can affect employment whilst illness itself and the ability to work to a previous pace may also result in job changes or curtailment. The loss of a job may ramify in terms of economic deprivation, social limitations, curtailed career and a loss of sense of purpose and ambition.

Family

HIV infection and AIDS have always been a disease that ramifies through the family. The family needs to be broadly interpreted (Miller and Bor 1989) and the effects on them can be dramatic, whether they are also infected or not.

Independence

HIV infection can challenge an individual's independence. Social, medical and financial reliance may increase as a direct or indirect result of infection.

LOSS AND AIDS-RELATED ILLNESSES

The natural history of HIV disease is marked by considerable periods of good health while the individual is HIV-positive and well. The extent of this period is poorly understood, and is documented to range from very short timespans to periods as long as knowledge about the virus has been available. An AIDS diagnosis occurs when specific opportunist infections occur. Again, the course of disease once an AIDS diagnosis has been made fluctuates dramatically. With the growing availability of interventions, prophylaxis and management, many conditions which were fatal early in the epidemic are now managed for considerable periods of time. The course of AIDS illness is thus punctuated by episodes of illness and good health. This phase can bring with it many emotional challenges. Unlike the period of HIV testing, diagnosis of an opportunistic infection equates an AIDS diagnosis. The way this is handled varies considerably. Some people are left to assume their changed status from HIV-positive to AIDS, whereas others may benefit from full dialogue and counselling.

AIDS may herald an additional set of losses which may include the following.

Active Health

The meandering course of AIDS-related illnesses may catapult an individual from phases of good health to life-threatening illness. The gaps and spaces between such episodes not only vary but are difficult in that they are unpredictable.

Freedom of Movement

AIDS may limit previous freedoms that may represent a poignant loss to an individual. Movement can be limited for a host of reasons ranging from discriminative entry requirements for certain countries, failing health, need for close proximity to medical carers, lack of motivation or energy, or fear of being too far away from home in case of illness or medication problems.

Independence

Much of the above may mark a loss of independence for an individual, which they can mourn with aching pain.

Self-image

One of the harshest losses experienced for an essentially young group of people relates to changes in body image, which can affect self-image dramatically. This can include excessive weight loss, hair loss due to certain treatments and skin marking due to conditions such as Kaposi's sarcoma. The problems need not be visible to affect self-image. Debilitating diarrhoea can be destructive to self-image, as can any number of mental constraints which change personality expression.

Decision Making

Some people are acutely distressed by a loss of freedom to make decisions or, on the other hand, the constant need to make decisions about their future, especially in the face of overwhelming uncertainty. People with AIDS may have many such situations. They may have to deliberate on treatment regimes, care regimes and life decisions. Some of the decisions are not straightforward, and there are no clear pathways.

FACING DEATH

Although every human will die, the knowledge that this is imminent can be traumatic and requires special focus. Death anxiety permeates the psyche of many individuals (Marcus and Rosenberg 1989) and may play a role in many psychological conditions. There is never certainty about death and workers should take great care not to make predictions and pronouncements for any individual. This needs to be weighed in careful balance with honesty and truth. When a person is clearly dying their enquiries need to be handled with candour, compassion and caring.

Hinton (1977) and Parkes (1986) have examined psychological aspects of dying in order to catalogue the areas that cause consternation to the dying. For example, in a survey of dying patients pain was often quoted as one of the greatest worries. However, in a study by Sherr and George (1987) people with AIDS were most likely to note 'telling others' as the cause of most concern. Besides being an indictment of society, such notions have implications for this disease, which is surrounded by social stigma.

There are a number of tasks that people who are facing death may want to contemplate. These may be done with ease for some, but with great difficulty for others. This results in a wide variety of individual reactions, where some people think through many of the issues, react and plan, while others do not take this on board, carry on very much in a day-to-day fashion, and leave some items unprepared. Both strategies (and all variations within the continuum) bring pain, difficulty and trauma. The kinds of tasks involved are discussed below.

Planning

There is a great deal of planning that can be associated with imminent death. This refers not only to mental and medical planning, but also to items such as writing of wills (Sherr 1989). Some people put off such tasks because they are concerned that any focus on wills may 'tempt fate' or trigger the onset of symptoms. Others may feel it is an admission of defeat. However, there are some individuals who glean much relief from the process of getting their affairs in order.

Intervention

Another task confronted by those facing dying concerns decisions about treatment, resuscitation and options. In Chapter 9 Alison Richardson goes into some detail about living wills (Eisendrath 1983). What is important in this task is often not the outcome, but the process itself. This can afford much anxiety relief and help an individual to have their thoughts, wishes and desires known. It also allows loved ones to follow these through, rather than face painful decisions on behalf of the dying which they may feel ill equipped to respond to.

Place

In the West many people die in hospital. However, new movements have been set up to facilitate a range of options regarding place of death. These can include hospital, hospice or home (Naysmith and O'Neill 1989). Decisions about place of terminal care are important and need to be backed up with realistic service provision. Hospice environments raise a number of specific questions for the dying, their close ones, the staff and for others at the hospice who may or may not witness dying. Honeybun, Johnston and Tookman (1992) compared a small group of patients who had shared a room with someone who had died with those who had not witnessed a death. Of interest was the consistent finding that those who had witnessed a death showed lower levels of depression. Indeed, these authors point out that such an experience was comforting rather than distressing. The implications for HIV-related death are clear, especially for individuals who may have concerns about the level of care and attendance they may expect. If they observe input to another they may certainly gain reassurance.

Symptoms

Dying may be associated with physical and psychological symptoms such as pain, breathlessness, fear, panic and sadness. Symptom control and reassurance should form part of all terminal care. This should extend to the loved ones surrounding the dying individual, who may themselves feel acute emotions and helplessness as they worry about their loved ones.

Closure

Closure is an important concept and embodies the notion of final farewells. Some people find it painful when those around the dying begin to disassociate, withdraw or retreat. Even when such closure cannot occur, symbolic closure can often play a vital role and allows much relief.

Creation of Memories

There are those who believe that grief is a process of forgetting and pushing away. However, psychological models would put forward an alternative view where grief is the process of finding a place and a form of expression for painful memories. A denial model would annihilate any memories, yet an incorporation model would encourage and acknowledge the need for memory creation. This may be particularly relevant if there are absent loved ones who may want to have some message or some clear memory of the dead.

Meaningful Lives

The pathway to death may be eased when people can balance meaningful lives into the equation. Help can come in the form of providing an occasion and facility to reflect on meaningful achievements, to highlight and commemorate these and to incorporate them into a sense of self worth.

The Dying Phase

The nature of death may not always be a downhill pathway. People may deteriorate and recuperate and they may need endless support as they move through these processes. When the terminal phase is reached, the dying individual needs constant, sensitive handling. Those around may be unused to the slow loss of physical ability and they should have constant contact with help sources, especially if the person has chosen to die at home. Panic and fear may be common as they see their loved one unable to breathe clearly or to communicate. Those attending the dying, especially if they have never done so before, may need some straightforward help.

GRIEF AFTER AN AIDS-RELATED DEATH

Death, whenever it comes, brings with it a finality and awesome realization. Immediately following a death there are a range of demands covering practical, emotional and life challenges. Worden (1991) provides a helpful analysis of mourning in terms of tasks. This allows for an observation of the tasks currently undertaken by the grieving and also allows for intervention if the grief-stricken become stuck on a certain task. Leick and Davidsen-Nielsen (1991) clarify how intervention can promote the acquisition of new skills to facilitate adapting to a new environment where the lost person is missing. Some authors examine alternating styles of connecting and disconnecting in AIDS bereavement experiences.

Practical Issues

At the very time when loved ones are confronted by a death, when they may be reeling from shock and disbelief, they are called upon to pace through some very practical events. Some people are able to do this with great clarity and composure, some find it monumentally difficult while others find the tasks themselves somewhat therapeutic. Indeed, many cultural norms about 'the way of death' seem to provide pacing and structure through the labyrinth of these very procedures. At a time when individuals may be stunned and uncertain, some find this clarity helpful while others find it difficult. Many of the cultural rituals serve similar purposes in terms of ensuring social support, relieving the bereaved of their daily duties, providing solace and action and allowing them to abdicate certain decisions. Workers involved with the bereaved need to acquaint themselves with the cultural rituals of their clients.

Other practical issues that need to be addressed include:

- Finance
- Legal formalities
- Burial formalities
- Cultural/religious issues.

THE SPECIAL BURDEN OF CARERS

No chapter on psychological issues surrounding death and bereavement is complete without comprehensive consideration of the needs of carers. There are a wide range of carers in AIDS and HIV disease. This is determined not only by the multidisciplinary nature of much of the formal care, but also by the unprecedented involvement of self-help and voluntary agencies as well as the high degree of involvement often shown by lovers, family and friends. If staff are exposed to the constant, unremitting death of people they care for, eventually they will find the burden awesomely difficult to bear. There is much evidence to show that good protocol, sensitive staff handling, provision of a wide range of support, and clear delineation of tasks may ameliorate these effects (see Bennett, Chapter 6 this volume).

Most health care workers report high levels of stress surrounding the death of a patient and interactions with both the patient and their family (Vachon 1987; Neimeyer 1988). Such anxiety may stem from the difficulty of such situations, from the feelings of personal vulnerability evoked by the situation or from the emotional pain engendered (Backer, Hannon and Russell 1982; Hines 1989; Ussher 1990). Parkes (1980, 1985) found that death and dying were major stressors for student nurses. This is often confounded by difficulties experienced by health care workers on how best to help those affected. Indeed, it is often noted that lowered mood can result from feelings of helplessness and this may well be a contributory factor for staff dealing with the dying and the bereaved. Burnout has often been discussed in challenging health care settings and death situations may well contribute to these. Firth, Cozens and Field (1991) tracked fear of death in a longitudinal cohort of medics and found fear greater for the dying than confronting someone who had already died. Yet coping strategies over time showed a move towards passive acceptance. They highlighted a gender difference, with male subjects more commonly resorting to rationalization techniques to accommodate the death and female subjects more likely to provide support for the patient (both clinically and emotionally). Of interest was the finding that fear and stress scores correlated with dismissal and avoidance.

Thus the literature tends to suggest that most professionals find coping with death a challenge. If no active strategies are evolved, fear and anxiety may heighten and this moves hand in hand with dismissal and avoidance. Such a situation must render workers of little help to the bereaved who are overwhelmed, confused, frightened and often inexperienced in the practicalities of death. Such knowledge is of interest when one notes that few workers have formal training for death-related work, let alone support in doing such work or debriefing and learning through the process. This has been a stark shortfall. Hines (1989) comments that it is invariably 'baptism by fire' where staff are thrown into a situation and often left alone to cope with any emotional reactions or turmoil.

Carers also include families. Most work is carried out on adults, yet children who are both affected and infected have specific needs. Chapters 10 and 12 set out in more detail some of the issues related to children. Halperin (1993) examined the role of denial in children whose parents died of AIDS. Dubik-Urruh and See (1989) describe some of the issues for dying children with dying families.

Normile (1990) compared psychological symptoms in the bereaved parents of adult children who died of cancer and those who died of AIDS ($n=58$). Parents bereaved by AIDS were significantly more depressed, anxious and exhibited higher obsessive–compulsive symptoms than parents bereaved by cancer. These authors found that grief was similar but that the parents of AIDS sufferers were characterized by greater somatization, depression and more intense overall distress, which may make them vulnerable to complicated grief and/or physical illness.

Myrick Torress (1989) compared the Kubler-Ross (1970) model in AIDS ($n = 30$) and cancer ($n = 30$) patients. People with AIDS became significantly more depressed than those with cancer. Anxieties related to death were significantly greater for the former group. People with AIDS showed greater depth of feeling whereas those with cancer were more likely to intellectualize and rationalize their condition. People with AIDS needed to talk about their losses while the cancer respondents analysed their grief. People with AIDS tended to indicate a greater need for family and peer support.

Lennon, Martin and Dean (1990) examined the relationships between instrumental and emotional social support and the experience of grief in 180 gay men who were bereaved of a lover or close friend due to AIDS in the early years of the epidemic. The findings showed that gay men losing a partner or friend reported similar symptoms of grief to those in studies of bereaved spouses and parents. Intensity of such grief reactions was influenced by caretaking during terminal phases of illness, and the perceived adequacy of social support. Emotional support during the course of the illness was associated with less intense symptoms of grief.

Some workers have documented post-traumatic stress and survivor problems in the AIDS bereaved (Colburn and Malena 1988; Ryan 1988; Trice 1988). Others have documented problems in the workplace and have examined the effects of bereavement on institutions that have been saturated by HIV related deaths that show no signs of respite. These authors urge for programmes to include education, resource development, time and acknowledgement of the loss if ongoing management is to be possible.

One of the historical facts of AIDS and HIV disease is the high level of support received from self-help groups. These are often staffed by individuals who themselves may be HIV-positive. This can compound the problems and great care must be taken to nourish such groups as they respond to the enormous toll of deaths left in the wake of HIV. As HIV is both sexually and transplacentally transmitted, there is often a familywide network of infection. Those who are bereaved may themselves be dying. Such a situation may result in a situation without precedent in the literature and much of the learning is gathered from experience.

THE BEREAVED

The bereaved in HIV disease have special requirements as they are often not only bereaved but facing HIV infection and illness themselves. Such individuals may have a qualitatively different experience and may have different hurdles, resources and reactions to those who are uninfected and bereaved.

Shock

The feelings of shock that are commonly described are experienced in a multitude of ways. They often include transient or elongated periods of being numb, inert, aloof, indifferent or detached.

Guilt

Acute anguish is an uncomfortable emotion that can be transitory or long-term. Guilt may surround mode of infection, recrimination about care and response, and negative feelings about level of commitment. Guilt can often interact when someone watches their loved one suffer and a side of them actively anticipates the end of such suffering. When it comes it may be hard to accommodate.

Survivor Syndrome

Survivor syndrome may well permeate the bereaved, especially if they have HIV-infected partners and have been exposed but have somehow escaped infection. Long-term survivors may also experience some of the emotions epitomized by this syndrome.

Niederlander (1981) describes an individual who after surviving a life-threatening situation presents with entrenched depression with resultant withdrawal and isolation. They may experience a wide range of symptoms that disturb them by intruding into memory, by reliving guilt and often via the experience of psychosomatic complaints. Intricate close relationships are key in the creation of self-validation. The loss, violation or abrupt termination of these leaves the bereaved not only saddened or decimated, but also adrift in terms of their own personal self-meaning. Survivor syndromes may have a particular impact on shattered worlds of meaning where identity becomes challenged and survivors may need external help to maintain self-preservation and cohesion.

Self-preservation

Marcus and Rosenberg (1989) discuss the importance of a frame of reference in the human pursuit of self-preservation and cohesion.

This concept can certainly exacerbate emotional bewilderment in the grief-stricken who lose a loved one, watch their peer group die and have to question their self-reference.

Going On

In the quest for continuation the bereaved often take stock of their life. They have to renegotiate a world without their loved one. They have to grapple with the fact that life goes on.

INTERVENTION

HIV infection heralds a host of 'bad news' incidents. One major intervention includes sensitizing and training staff to handle such situations. Psychological or counselling models may be particularly helpful in this regard. Although counselling cannot remove the experience of bad news, it can be used to ensure that the news is given in the best way possible. Giving bad news is a difficult task. Again, without training, the pain of such a procedure may often result in a withdrawing profession. Such withdrawal is the inevitable strategy of protection for those who are not helped. Indeed, many professional boundaries and barriers have evolved to facilitate such withdrawal.

All skill acquisition can be achieved by a variety of means. These include formal training, experience, practice and video feedback. If training is not provided then learning occurs from experience (often including role modelling where a previously untrained superior is imitated, irrespective of their skill at the task). Such a method is risky as bad practice can multiply.

Breaking news forms part of the communication aspect of medical inter-actions. Reviews of the literature on patient satisfaction (see, for example, Ley 1988) have recorded a consistent dissatisfaction with communication aspects of care. Furthermore, with training these aspects can be improved. Given that such literature exists, it could be seen now as poor practice if suitable training is withheld. Indeed, many medical schools now include communication training in their curriculum.

TALKING TO THE DYING

The medical model is concerned with cure, but people with AIDS often need care where no cure is available. The complexities of AIDS illnesses often involve a myriad of experts. This can leave the individual behind.

Emotional support may be packaged off and sent to psychologists (Ussher 1990) who themselves may be ill equipped to provide magic answers. Yet the counselling model may allow for an approach which supplements medical care and is the only way forward in the absence of a cure. This means that the individual should have the opportunity as well as the right to consider their emotions and needs and have these responded to. There is no literature helpful in determining how one should talk to the dying. Yet clearly the message for all workers is 'talk to the dying'. This does not necessarily have to be talk about death. Indeed, many AIDS patients are barraged by well meaning carers who want to discuss their death while they would prefer to discuss living.

Some factual information is invariably desired. Indeed, the majority of studies with other groups of dying patients show, in general, that people would like to know of their impending death, although this dialogue is often not forthcoming (Kalish 1978; Wilson 1989). Studies have shown that people who are dying know this (Hinton 1963; Kubler-Ross 1970; Cartright, Hockey and Anderson 1973). Differential coping with such knowledge has been described by Hinton (1984). People vary, with some denying the death and others eager to gather as much knowledge and insight as possible.

Work with the dying must acknowledge a potential for psychological disturbance, which has been described either directly as a result of dying or indirectly as a response to treatments (Peck and Boland 1977; Forester, Kornfield and Fleiss, 1978). This is not inevitable as Hinton and Forester both document low levels of disturbance in individuals who had previous high levels of coping in stressful situations and Silberfarb, Maurer and Crowthamel (1980) caution against misinterpreting signs of illness as somatic signs of depression. The major problems noted include anxiety, depression and confusion.

Devise a Substitute

Sometimes this is embodied by work in HIV and AIDS organizations, dedication to a cause or rebuilding memories. It provides a focus for energy, pain and an ability to create some form of internal and external meaning. Command and control can also be reintroduced to a survivor who previously felt at a loss, out of control and unable to master the course of disease in someone they not only cared for but that they thought would survive for many years to come.

Trust

The death may prompt a sense of abandonment so painful that the thought of commencing a new relationship is almost unthinkable; tasks are centred around slowly building up a new framework and new links with humanity.

Visions and Concepts

Help comes in the form of allowing the person to weave their experience into a whole, placing together the negative events of the death with life events. This will allow them to view living much more broadly and to look forward to possible enjoyment rather than to remain stuck and narrowly focused onto the negative and traumatic events.

Expression of Grief

The expression of grief by an individual can take many varied forms. Worden (1991) points out that one of the 'tasks' of grief may be the need to experience the pain of grief. Leick and Davidsen-Nielsen (1991) point out the utility of detailed incident recounting, letter writing and the use of memorabilia (such as photographs, music or cherished objects) to prompt visions and detailed recall.

The experience of grief can be aided by self-help and support groups. In extreme situations intervention from more intensive sources can be necessary.

Non-resolution of Grief

Although it is difficult to describe true resolution, there is a considerable literature on problems that occur surrounding grief. Schuchter and Zisook (1993) summarize it as follows:

- Atypical (Parkes 1972)
- Morbid (Lindemann 1944)
- Pathological (Volkan 1972; Raphael 1975; Middleton et al 1993)
- Absent (Deutsch 1937)
- Abnormal (Hackett 1974)
- Neurotic (Wahl 1970)
- Depressive (Clayton, Halikar and Maurice 1972).

Detailed examinations of such grief-related problems are summarized by Catalan in Chapter 4, this volume. Predictors or risk factors for problems are reported in conditions where:

- Social support is weak or lacking
- There is a pre-existing history of psychiatric conditions, notably mood disorders
- Grief occurs simultaneously with other traumatic life events

- The bereaved themselves are ill
- The bereavement heralds multiple changes, such as financial loss, housing loss, support loss
- The relationship was excessively intimate
- The relationship was highly dependent
- The relationship was typified by friction or discord
- The relationship was typified by ambivalence.

Leick and Davidsen-Neilsen (1991) set out risk factors for pathological grief. These include:

- The circumstances surrounding the loss
- The personality of the mourner
- The nature and extent of attachment to the lost person
- The psychological situation of the mourner.

Unfortunately the very nature of AIDS and HIV infection often triggers many of the above to occur simultaneously. As AIDS itself is sexually transmitted, there is a possibility that loved ones are also infected, thus facing concurrent life events, perhaps illness, change of economic and social circumstance and fluctuations in intensity and nature of relationships. The stigma that is often associated with HIV infection and AIDS may further alienate and isolate the grieving. Confidentiality and avoidance issues may hinder pathways of support and an overreliance on health care professionals may render support inadequate or not of the quality which is meaningful and useful to the bereaved.

Disengagement

Disengagement is a process that can frequently be observed. Once an individual enters the terminal phase of an illness and death appears imminent, those surrounding them find it difficult to engage and approach the dying person. Often this relates to their own fears and confusion. Efforts should be made to overcome this. Many of the mainstream interventions utilized by psychologists are relevant for work with the dying, including anxiety and depression management, and facilitation of open feelings (Wilson 1989).

CAUSES FOR CONCERN

Although HIV and AIDS are relatively new, there is no reason to presume that the growing body of knowledge on grief and bereavement should not be relevant to this group, given adjustment for individual differences and illness factors. A series of issues has been shown to be associated with possible problems in other areas. They bear consideration in relation to AIDS and HIV.

Immune Functioning

There are some workers who have catalogued changes in immune function coinciding with bereavement (Irwin and Pike 1993). The nature and mechanisms of such a link are still unclear, but may potentially have a negative impact in AIDS-related bereavement. As HIV is sexually transmitted and an immune-compromising disorder, there is an increased likelihood that the bereaved will be HIV-positive and will also be sensitive to any immune-compromising conditions.

Bereavement Outcome Risk Factors

Sanders (1993) has summarized a range of risk factors which may necessitate intervention. No text on bereavement should fail to point out the high risks, both in terms of mental and physical health, to the survivors. AIDS and HIV infection lend themselves to many of the categories of risk outlined by Sanders.

Age

Younger individuals have been shown to have higher intensity of reaction in grief (Ball 1977; Sanders 1981). AIDS and HIV infection disproportionately affect the young.

Gender

The data on gender are ambiguous. Most studies show that bereaved men fare less well. This may be accounted for by a variety of explanations including social support, differential symptom experience and reporting, and differential help seeking. However, there are specific gender-related issues associated with AIDS and HIV infection, and care should be taken to promote current support and self-help groups and to facilitate access to such support.

Parental Grief

Sanders notes that mothers grieve more intensely than fathers, yet there is a paucity of literature on the subject. HIV-related infant deaths may bring with them a specific form of grief, especially if infection was vertical and parents are suffering under the dual burden of personal infection and child loss.

Reduced Material Resources

Poor adjustment in bereavement is compounded by poverty (Jacobs et al 1989). AIDS and HIV infection may be directly linked with limited material resources. Ignorance and discrimination are rife and unemployment is not uncommon. The burden of AIDS caring may make work and regular employment difficult. This may also be hindered by the oscillating nature of AIDS-related illnesses. The cumulative result may well be reduced material resources for the dying and the bereaved.

Personality

Sanders notes that there are a multitude of personality factors that may affect bereavement reaction or predispose individuals to specific outcomes. The research literature is deficient in this area. In terms of intervention there is a clear need to react with flexibility to the wide range of personality factors associated with the individuals who are affected. Particular issues of note refer to ambivalence and dependency. Both these notions may well be present in an AIDS-related bereavement.

Health Prior to Bereavement

Pre-existing health may play a key role in the strength and stamina with which the bereaved face their new life circumstance. If the bereaved are themselves HIV-positive they may well be challenged and in need of high levels of support.

Stigmatized Death

The bereaved may have to face a double burden. The first is that associated with the loss, and the second is associated with the stigma. AIDS is a highly stigmatized condition and the bereaved who survive an AIDS-related death may be cut off from their natural grieving process by hurdles created by the stigma or by their need for subterfuge and lies to counterbalance the stigma.

Mode of Death

Marzuk and colleagues (1988) have shown an increased suicide risk for people with AIDS. There is a divided opinion in the literature on the risks faced by the bereaved if death was as a result of suicide (Osterweis, Solomon and Green 1984; Wrobliski and McIntosh 1987).

Social Support

There is a considerable body of literature that points to the key role of social support and the associated problems when this commodity is lacking (Ostrow 1990; Green 1993). AIDS and HIV infection often alienate individuals and are sometimes related to strained social support. This situation may well be exacerbated by the multiple nature of bereavement. When support agencies and self-help groups are themselves strained by continued losses social support networks may be dramatically challenged.

Parallel Crises

Sanders notes that concurrent crises may be a risk factor. The likelihood of parallel crises for someone bereaved by AIDS is high. AIDS and HIV differ in many respects from other infections. By the very nature of the virus, infection is often multiple and there may be many members of communities, families and networks who are affected and infected. Furthermore, in many communities AIDS does not mark a single isolated death, but ravages the community whereby individuals suffer from multiple loss (Sherr et al 1992). The only comparable literature where analogous examples can be gleaned is that on situations of multiple death, such as war or disaster. In war literature multiple exposure to deaths is often associated with a numbing effect. No such effect has been noted in AIDS (Sherr et al 1992). Multiple bereavement may enhance the burden of grief for those who are continuously exposed and at times also have deteriorating health themselves.

Suicide and Parasuicide

AIDS and HIV infection are associated with an increased likelihood of suicide (Marzuk et al 1988; Brown and Rundell 1989; Plott, Benton and Winslade 1989; Atkinson et al 1990; Kathke 1991; Cote, Biggar and Dannenberg 1992), which is reported as 36 times greater in some studies (Marzuk et al 1988). Suicide trends in general are a cause for grave concern (Davidson 1989). Many explanations still revolve around the early classifications of Durkheim (1897). Suicide associated issues manifest in many forms ranging from ideation, attempts, completed acts and associated bereavement. Suicidal thoughts and acts in association with HIV disease tend to concentrate around the time of diagnosis and again at end stage disease. There is also a worrying association between HIV testing and suicide ideation (Perry, Jacobsberg and Fisham 1990; Neugebauer and Johnson 1990).

The general literature points to specific bereavement hurdles for those surviving a suicide. Bereavement itself has been associated with suicide (Bunch 1972). The effects of suicide on the nature and experience of grief in HIV disease are relatively uncharted and will become apparent as the epidemic unfolds (Flavin et al 1986).

Suicidal problems in HIV disease may differ systematically for those in the two peak periods. The trauma of early diagnosis and infection may trigger suicidal ideation or acts for some. This may be associated with the way in which testing was carried out, support at the time, individual ability to cope, social support and emotional resources. At late stage illness, suicide options are considered and encountered by some. The reasons and triggers are complex and probably vary from individual to individual (Gutierrez et al 1990; Papathomopoulos 1988). Many individuals at end stage disease question the quality of their life and the ability to control, at least, their right to die. This raises a wide range of ethical, moral and practical questions, particularly addressed in studies from the Netherlands where euthanasia is reported (Van den Boom et al 1991).

Very often the burden of life in the presence of HIV is difficult to bear. Service provision may be inadequate and challenge staff dramatically (Slome et al 1990). Suicidal acts are certainly a form of taking control for some individuals who feel that control in many other spheres is elusive in the presence of HIV. Those whose loved ones die as a result of suicide may be particularly vulnerable. If they themselves are HIV positive this effect may be enhanced.

CONCLUSIONS

Why is AIDS such a taboo subject? Could it be that it sweeps into its arena every previously held taboo of mankind such as sex, sexuality, blood and drugs? Or does it provide a double taboo which is so enormous that few are able to challenge it honestly? The double taboo is one where the subject of death cannot be avoided and the pain of the living cut down so arbitrarily can either be faced or, as is the usual reaction to death, ignored, evaded, removed or sanitized. AIDS is unavoidably linked with death (Ussher 1990), the fear or anticipation thereof (Sherr 1989) and the confrontation of bereavement, often on a massive scale (Dean, Hall and Martin 1988; McCusick 1991). Yet there is much that can be done for the dying and bereaved irrespective of whether life can be saved or not. When questioned many people do not fear 'being dead' but fear 'dying'. The process of helping people around dying is one where they are essentially viewed as living. Training prior to exposure may help workers to accommodate to many of the difficult challenges posed by the multitude of deaths left in the wake of AIDS. Failure to address the issues may result in disengagement, estrangement, excessive stress and burnout. Carers suffering from these may well provide shallow interactions and poor quality of care.

REFERENCES

Atkinson H, Gutierrez R, Cottler L et al (1990) Suicide ideation and attempts in HIV illness *VI Int AIDS Conf* (San Francisco) Abstr SB 384

Backer BA, Hannon N & Russell NA (1982) *Death and Dying: Individuals and Institutions* New York: Wiley

Ball J (1977) Widow's grief: the impact of age and mode of death *Omega* **7**: 307–33

Beckenridge J, Gallagher D, Thompson L & Peterson J (1986) Characteristic depressive symptoms of bereaved elders *J Gerontol* **41**: 163–8

Bornstein P, Clayton P, Halikas J et al (1973) The depression of widowhood after 13 months *Br J Psychiatry* **122**: 561–6

Brown GR & Rundell JR (1989) Suicidal tendencies in women with human immunodeficiency virus infection *Am J Psychiatry* **146**(4): 556–7

Bunch J (1972) Recent bereavement in relation to suicide *J Psychosom Res* **16**: 361–6

Burren Van HJ, Lunter C, Van Den Boom F & Storosum J (1991) Prevalence of psychiatric and psychosocial complications among HIV infected patients in the Netherlands *VII Int AIDS Conf* Abstr MB 2104

Cartright A, Hockey L & Anderson J (1973) *Life before Death* London: Routledge and Kegan Paul

Clayton P, Halikas J & Maurice W (1972) The depression of widowhood *Br J Psychiatry* **120**: 71–6

Colburn KA & Malena D (1988) Bereavement issues for survivors of persons with AIDS: coping with society's pressures *Am J Hosp Care* **5**: 20–5

Cote T, Biggar K & Dannenberg A (1992) Risk of suicide among PWA *JAMA* **268**(15): 2066–8

Davidson S (1989) Suicide. In L Sherr (ed) *Death, Dying and Bereavement* Oxford: Blackwell Scientific pp 215–241

Dean L, Hall WE & Martin JL (1988) Chronic and intermittent AIDS-related bereavement in a panel of homosexual men in New York City *J Palliat Care* **4**: 54–7

Deutsch H (1937) Absence of grief *Psychoanal Q* **6**: 12–22

Dubik-Urruh S & See V (1989) Children of chaos: planning for the emotional survival of dying children of dying families *J Palliat Care* **5**: 10–15

Durkheim E (1897) *Suicide, a Study of Sociology* (trans. JA Spaulding & G Simpson, 1951) New York: Free Press

Eisendrath F (1983) The living will: help or hindrance? *JAMA* **249**: 2054–8

Firth Cozens J & Field D (1991) Fear of death and strategies for coping with patient death among medical trainees *Br J Med Psychol* **64**: 263–71

Flavin DK, Franklin JE & Frances RJ (1986) The acquired immune deficiency syndrome, AIDS, and suicidal behaviour in alcohol-dependent homosexual men. *Am J Psychiatry* **143**: 1440–2

Forester B, Kornfield M & Fleiss J (1978) Psychiatric aspects of radiotherapy *Am J Psychiatry* **135**: 960–3

Frances RJ, Wikstrom T & Alcena V (1985) Contracting AIDS as a means of committing suicide *Am J Psychiatry* **142**: 656

Goin M, Burgoyne R & Goin J (1979) Timeless attachment to a dead relative *Am J Psychiatry* **136**: 988–9

Green G (1993) Social support and HIV *AIDS Care* **5**(3): 87–104

Green J & Sherr L (1989) Dying, bereavement and loss. In J Green & A McCreaner (eds) *Counselling in HIV Infection and AIDS* Oxford: Blackwell Scientific pp 207–23

Gutierrez R, Atkinson H, Velin R et al (1990) Coping and neuropsychological correlates of suicidality in HIV *VI Int AIDS Conf* (San Francisco) Abstr SB 386

Hackett T (1974) Recognizing and treating abnormal grief *Hosp Physician* **1**: 49–54

Halperin E (1993) Denial in children whose parents died of AIDS *Child Psychiatry Hum Dev* **4**: 249–57

Hines N (1989) Care for the carers. In L Sherr (ed) *Death, Dying and Bereavement* Oxford: Blackwell Scientific pp 78–92

Hinton J (1963) The physical and mental distress of the dying *Q J Med* **32**: 1–21

Hinton J (1977) *Dying* London: Penguin

Hinton J (1984) Coping with terminal illness. In J Fitzpatrick, JM Hinton, S Newman et al (eds) *The Experience of Illness* London: Tavistock Publications pp 227–45

Honeybun J, Johnston M & Tookman A (1992) The impact of death on fellow hospice patients *Br J Med Psychol* **65**: 67–72

House J (1981) *Work Stress and Social Support* Reading: Addison-Wesley

Irwin M & Pike J (1993) Bereavement, depressive symptoms and immune function. In M Stroebe, W Stroebe & R Hansson (eds) *Handbook of Bereavement* Cambridge: Cambridge University Press pp 160–74

Jacobs S, Hansen F, Berkman L et al (1989) Depressions of bereavement *Compr Psychiatry* **30**: 218–24

Jennet B (1987) Conference: decisions to limit treatment *Lancet* ii: 787–9

Kalish R (1978) A little myth is a dangerous thing: research in the service of the dying. In CA Garfield (ed) *Psychological Care of the Dying Patient* New York: McGraw Hill

Karlinsky H, Taerk G, Schwartz K et al (1988) Suicide attempts and resuscitation dilemmas *Gen Hosp Psychiatry* **10**: 423–30

Kathke N (1991) Cases of unnatural death and AIDS-related death in Munich *AIDS Forschung* **8**: 11–16

Kubler-Ross E (1970) *On Death and Dying* London: Macmillan

Leick N & Davidsen-Nielsen M (1991) *Healing Pain – Attachment Loss and Grief Therapy* London: Routledge

Lennon MC, Martin JL & Dean L (1990) The influence of social support on AIDS-related grief reaction among gay men *Soc Sci Med* **31**: 477–84

Ley P (1988) *Communicating with Patients: Improving Communication, Satisfaction and Compliance*. London: Croom Helm.

Lindemann E (1944) Symptomatology and management of acute grief *Am J Psychiatry* **101**: 141–8

Lynn J (1989) Correspondence *N Engl J Med* **321**: 119–20

McCann K & Wadsworth E (1991) The experience of having a positive HIV antibody test *AIDS Care* **3**: 43–54

McCusick L (1990) Plenary Address *VII Int AIDS Conf* (Florence)

Marcus P & Rosenberg A (1989) Survivors of man-made mass death. In L Sherr (ed) *Death, Dying and Bereavement* Oxford: Blackwell Scientific pp 122–45

Marzuk PM, Tierney H, Tardiff K et al (1988) Increased risk of suicide in persons with AIDS *JAMA* **259**: 1333–7

Middleton W, Raphael B, Martinek N & Misso V (1993) Pathological grief reactions. In M Stroebe, W Stroebe & R Hansson (eds) *Handbook of Bereavement* Cambridge: Cambridge University Press pp 44–61

Miller D (1990) Diagnosis and treatment of acute psychological problems related to HIV infection and disease. In D Ostrow (ed) *Behavioral Aspects of AIDS* New York: Plenum Medical pp 187–204

Miller R & Bor R (1989) *AIDS, a Guide to Clinical Counselling* London: Science Press

Myrick Torress JJ (1989) Grief process: the relationship between AIDS patients and cancer patients *Diss Abstr Int B* **50**: 1639

Natterson J & Knudson A (1960) Observations concerning fear of death in fatally ill children and their mothers *Psychosom Med* **22**: 465

Naysmith A & O'Neill W (1989) Hospice. In L Sherr (ed) *Death Dying and Bereavement* Oxford: Blackwell Scientific pp 1–16

Neimeyer RA (1988) Death anxiety. In H Wass, FM Berado & RA Neimeyer (eds) *Dying: Facing the Facts* (2nd edn) Washington: Hemisphere

Neugebauer R & Johnson J (1990) Does HIV testing raise levels of suicidal ideation? *JAMA* **263**: 679–82

Niederlander W (1981) The survivor syndrome: further observations and dimensions *J Am Psychoanal Assoc* **29**: 413–26

Normile LB (1990) Psychological distress in bereavement: a comparative study of parents of adult children who died of cancer versus AIDS *Diss Abstr Int B* **50**: 2840

Osterweis M, Solomon F & Green M (1984) *Bereavement Reactions Consequences and Care* Washington: National Academy Press

Ostrow D (1990) *Behavioral Aspects of AIDS* New York: Plenum Medical

Papathomopoulos E (1988) An attempt to commit suicide by contracting AIDS *Am J Psychiatry* **145**: 765–6

Parga FJ (1989) Suicidal thoughts and acts in HIV infection suspects *V Int AIDS Conf* (Montreal) Abstr D 676

Parkes CM (1971) The first year of bereavement. A longitudinal study of the reaction of London widows to the death of their husbands *Psychiatry* **33**: 444–66

Parkes CM (1972) *Bereavement Studies of Grief in Adult Life* 2nd edn New York: International University Press

Parkes CM (1986) *Bereavement* (2nd edn) London: Pelican

Parkes CM (1993) Bereavement as a psychosocial transition: processes of adaptation to change. In M Stroebe, W Stroebe & R Hansson (eds) *Handbook of Bereavement* Cambridge: Cambridge University Press pp 91–101

Parkes K (1980) Occupational stress among student nurses *Nursing Times* **76**: 113–19

Parkes K (1985) Stressful episodes reported by first year student nurses. A descriptive account *Soc Sci Med* **20**: 945–53

Parkes CM & Weiss RS (1983) *Recovery from Bereavement* New York: Basic Books

Peck A & Boland J (1977) Emotional reactions to radiation treatment *Cancer* **40**: 180–4

Perry S, Jacobsberg L & Fishman B (1990) Suicidal ideation and HIV testing *JAMA* **263**: 679–92

Plott RT, Benton SD & Winslade WJ (1989) Suicide of AIDS patients in Texas: A preliminary report *Tex Med* **85**: 40–3

Raphael B (1975) The management of pathological grief *Aust N Z J Psychiatry* **9**: 173–80

Rook K (1987) Social support versus companionship: effects on life stress, loneliness and evaluations by others *J Pers Soc Psychol* **52**: 1132–47

Ryan MS (1988) Neglected survivors *Am J Nurs* **88**: 1070

Sanders C (1981) Comparisons of younger and older spouses in bereavement outcome *Omega* **11**: 217–32

Sanders C (1983) Effects of sudden versus chronic illness death on bereavement outcome *Omega* **11**: 227–41

Sanders C (1993) Risk factors in bereavement outcome. In M Stroebe, W Stroebe & R Hansson (eds) *Handbook of Bereavement* Cambridge: Cambridge University Press pp 255–70

Schilling RF (1987) Limitations of social support *Social Service Review* **61**: 16–31

Schneidman ES (1976) Suicide. In AM Freedman, HI Kaplan & BJ Sadock (eds) *Comprehensive Textbook of Psychiatry* Baltimore: Williams and Wilkins

Schuchter S & Zisook S (1993) The course of normal grief. In M Stroebe, W Stroebe & R Hansson (eds) *Handbook of Bereavement* Cambridge: Cambridge University Press pp 23–43

Sherr L (1989) *Death, Dying and Bereavement* Oxford: Blackwell Scientific

Sherr L & Davey T (1990) Counselling implications of anxiety and depression in AIDS and HIV infection: a pilot study *Counselling Psychol Q* **4**: 27–35

Sherr L, George H (1987) Staff support and HIV. Paper presented at Int Health Psychol Conf (Wales)

Sherr L & George H (1989) Loss and the human immunodeficiency virus. In L Sherr (ed) *Death, Dying and Bereavement* Oxford: Blackwell Scientific pp 161–78

Sherr L, Hedge B, Steinhart K et al (1992) Unique patterns of bereavement in HIV: implications for counselling *Genitourin Med* **82**: 68

Sherr L, Petrak J, Melvin D et al (1993) Psychological trauma associated with AIDS and HIV infection in women *Counselling Psychol Q* **6**: 99–108

Silberfarb P, Maurer H & Crowthamel C (1980) Psychosocial aspects of neoplastic disease. Functional status of breast cancer patients during different treatment regimes *Am J Psychiatry* **137**: 450–5

Slome LR, Moulton JM, Huffine C et al (1990) Physicians' attitudes toward assisted suicide in AIDS *VI Int AIDS Conf* (San Francisco) Abstr SD 858

Stroebe M, Stroebe W & Hansson R (1993) *Handbook of Bereavement* Cambridge: Cambridge University Press

Stroebe W & Stroebe M (1987) *Bereavement and Health* New York: Cambridge University Press

Thoits PA (1985) Social support and psychological well-being: theoretical possibilities. In IG Sarason & BR Sarason (eds) *Social Support Theory Research and Application* Dordrecht: Martinus Nijhoff pp 51–72

Trice AD (1988) Posttraumatic stress syndrome-like symptoms among AIDS caregivers *Psychol Rep* **63**: 656–8

Ussher J (1990) Professionals don't cry: death and dying in AIDS psychology *Changes* **8**: 284–93

Vachon M (1987) *Occupational Stress in Caring for the Critically Ill, the Dying and the Bereaved* Washington: Hemisphere

Van Den Boom F, Mead C, Grennen T & Roozenburg H (1991) AIDS, euthanasia and grief *VII Int AIDS Conf* (Florence) Abstr MD55

Volkan V (1972) The recognition and prevention of pathological grief *Va Med Monthly* **99**: 535–40

Wahl C (1970) The differential diagnosis of normal and neurotic grief following bereavement *Psychosomatics* **11**: 104–6

Wethington F & Kesler R (1986) Perceived support, received support and adjustment to stressful life events *J Hlth Soc Behav* **27**: 78–89

Wilson C (1989) Terminal care. In AK Broome (ed) *Health Psychology Processes and Applications* London: Chapman and Hall pp 405–18

Worden JW (1991) *Grief Counselling and Grief Therapy* London: Routledge

Wrobliski A & McIntosh J (1987) Problems of suicide survivors. A survey report *Isr J Psychiatry Relat Sci* **24**: 137–42

CHAPTER 2

The Epidemiology and Impact of AIDS-Related Death and Dying in New York's Gay Community

Laura Dean

*Columbia University in the City of New York,
New York, USA*

THE AIDS EPIDEMIC

AIDS (acquired immune deficiency syndrome), a fatal disease first detected in homosexual men living in New York City, Los Angeles and San Francisco in 1981, has ravaged our cities. Nowhere is this more true than in the gay communities of the Western world. In the United States alone over 130 000 cases of AIDS had been reported to the Centers for Disease Control (CDC) by the end of 1991. The majority (77%) of those diagnosed were dead (CDC 1993). Included in these totals are 19 500 gay men from New York City (New York City Department of Health Office of AIDS Surveillance 1993a). These figures do not, however, include the many gay men infected with HIV (human immunodeficiency virus), the cause of AIDS, who have not been diagnosed with the disease.

Estimates of HIV seroprevalence among gay men in New York City have ranged from 36% to 67%. The variability in estimates is clearly related to the sampling source and the purposes of the study. The lowest estimate of 36% comes from tests of adult men enrolled from diverse channels (excluding AIDS organizations and clinics) to determine the psychological impact of AIDS on the gay community (Martin, Dean, Garcia and Hall 1989),

Grief and AIDS. Edited by L. Sherr.
©1995 John Wiley & Sons Ltd.

a larger estimate of 44% is derived from tests of men who were participants in the hepatitis-B vaccine trials (Stevens et al 1986), and the highest estimate of 67% is based on a study of gay men recruited from health clinics (Curran et al 1985).

AIDS cases surged in New York's gay community in the early 1980s. Since 1985 an average of 2300 new cases have been diagnosed in each year (New York City Department of Health, Office of AIDS Surveillance 1993b). Media reports of the increasing AIDS cases in other high-risk groups have given some the erroneous impression that the AIDS epidemic is over in the gay community. Though annual AIDS case rates among gay men have not grown at the same rate in the later years of the epidemic as they did in earlier years, the diagnoses of AIDS cases have not abated. Approximately six New York City gay men are newly diagnosed each day, and while people with a diagnosis of AIDS are living longer due to earlier diagnosis, pneumocystis pneumonia (PCP) prophylaxis and zidovudine therapy, the deaths due to the disease continue.

THE STUDY OF DEATH AND DYING

AIDS has enveloped gay communities, creating in essence laboratories for the long-term study of the effects of death and dying in the young. Individuals from a wide range of disciplines – the helping professions (law, ethics, social work, nursing, public health, psychology, medicine), the biological and social sciences, the humanities and the arts – have all added to the discussion of this topic. Clinicians riveted by their experiences working with AIDS patients, their families and friends, have codified their impressions, written case studies, and described the process of dying and their reactions to it. Handbooks, guides, newsletters and bibliographies for people with AIDS and the AIDS-bereaved and their counselors have been published. Students have turned their attention to the topic and masters' theses and doctoral dissertations have been completed and archived.

An outpouring of journalistic and artistic renderings in response to the epidemic has appeared. Many of the works documenting the impact of death and dying are legacies from members of the gay community, many of whom were – or are – themselves afflicted with AIDS. The proliferation of these poignant works is in fact an indicator of the psychological impact of AIDS, and the writings are cathartic for those who grieve.

Little, however, is systematically known about either the breadth or depth of AIDS-related bereavement and grief, and there are few carefully designed, theoretically driven research studies of the subject. Our ongoing work on the epidemiology and psychosocial correlates of AIDS-related bereavement in New York's gay community is an attempt to bridge that gap. Here I will update an earlier review (Martin and Dean 1993b) of findings from completed analyses. There are characteristics of the stages of HIV illness which make AIDS deaths and bereavement unique, especially in relation to the gay community in which so many AIDS deaths have already occurred.

HIV Progression

There is evidence to show that how a person dies influences the subsequent psychosocial adjustment of survivors (see Stroebe and Stroebe 1987: 204–15). While AIDS deaths are like those from other chronic debilitating illnesses in many ways, they are also unique in important ways. In his popular book *How We Die*, Nuland (1994: 183–93) describes the course that HIV takes after entering a new host. The virus is transmitted either (1) through exposure to contaminated blood, (2) from an infected pregnant woman to her unborn child, or (3) through sexual intercourse with an infected partner. After infection the virus replicates rapidly, and its concentration in the blood is very high for two to four weeks. During this period some people develop a flu-like syndrome, ending with the first appearance of antibodies against HIV. The body successfully fights off the first massive number of virus particles that are produced, their concentration in the blood is stabilized and the microbes hide in the CD4 helper lymphocytes, lymph nodes, bone marrow, the central nervous system and spleen. Substantial damage to the immune system occurs during this clinically quiescent phase of the disease. After this period, which lasts from three to ten years, blood tests will indicate that CD4 cells have declined precipitously, from a normal count of 800–1200 per cubic millimeter to less than 400.

In about 18 months, skin tests for allergy will indicate that the immune system is impaired. Although the course is variable and some individuals will not yet show signs of clinical illness, most infected individuals will develop oral fungal infections after CD4 cell counts have fallen below 300. Additional infections, including non-specific indicators of disease such as fever, weight loss, fatigue, diarrhea and skin problems, may also appear. After the CD4 cell count declines to 200 there is an increased vulnerability to opportunistic infections beyond the skin and orifices. One reaches full-blown AIDS (CDC 1992) at this point, as the body is invaded by an array of deadly diseases such as pneumocystis pneumonia and Kaposi's sarcoma. These opportunistic diseases cannot be combated by a depleted immune system and only a minority of individuals survive for two years after diagnosis.

The illness, which develops over a long period of time, leads to increasing debilities and increasing demands for emotional and concrete support from others. The illness eventually results in lost role functioning at home and work, the diminution of sensory pleasures, and a reduction in or elimination of social involvement. Material hardship may result from either loss of income or insurance and exorbitant medical costs. Two characteristics of AIDS may be important in understanding grief reactions following AIDS bereavement: the first is the long period of anticipation of death, and the second is the harsh and often humiliating course of the disease.

During the first five years of the epidemic the period of asymptomatic infection was not considered part of the disease. The cause of AIDS was unknown and the means to detect infection were unavailable. However, with the discovery of HIV, the availability of reliable HIV antibody tests, and publicly funded blood-testing facilities, any individual wishing to know their infection status may now avail themselves of that information. The period of asymptomatic HIV infection may be an important time not only for anticipating death but also for engaging in hopefulness and adaptive denial (Folkman 1993). This is true for both the infected individual and those close to them. With the development of symptoms one reaches a new stage of adaptation. While the period of being clinically ill with AIDS has extended somewhat due to treatment, it is still extremely rare to survive five years after diagnosis with AIDS. This period of anticipatory dread may not ease the impact of the loss: death due to AIDS is not usually a quiet or peaceful process. People with AIDS and their caregivers often engage in intensive fights for life. The natural course of the illness is characterized by alterations between relatively normal daily functioning and serious disability, until death occurs either from the treatment, suicide or disease processes. The opportunistic infections and cancers associated with advancing AIDS are frequently painful and often disfiguring. Diagnostic procedures and treatments, as well as the illnesses themselves, often result in nausea, fever, incontinence and wasting. Thus, the lengthy time of anticipating death during the later stage of AIDS may be so traumatic that any buffering or adaptive function of the anticipatory period may be lost.

The emotions aroused during the period of caring for someone with AIDS may be intensely distressing. It is not unusual for both the person with AIDS and their caretakers to prefer death over life with AIDS. Wishing for the death of a loved one, or assisting with suicide, no matter how humane, can be the source of serious pain or guilt, complicating bereavement reactions.

While AIDS deaths share similarities to death from other causes, AIDS is also special. Unlike most degenerative diseases, AIDS strikes young to middle-aged adults in the prime of life, many of whom are at their peak of productivity. The occurrence of premature death can lead to greater intensity of grief reactions and increase the risk of prolonged or pathological grief outcomes (Lopata 1979; Parkes and Weiss 1983).

AIDS is also a stigmatizing illness, for both the person who is sick as well as those close to him (Sontag 1989; Herek 1991). AIDS has forced into the open some men's sexual identity. In some cases this forced 'outing' has improved relationships with others, but for many it has been very stressful. Irrational fears about contagion and the lack of understanding of AIDS, even among health care workers, add additional layers of strain for those who attempt to keep their dignity through the course of illness and death.

In addition to these unique characteristics of the disease, the community context in which AIDS flourishes makes AIDS bereavement among gay men special when compared with bereavement from other causes in other groups. The epidemic appeared first in a community possessing both organizational skills and material resources (Altman 1986; Shilts 1987). The people most involved in trying to control the epidemic and care for the sick constitute the group at highest risk of succumbing to the illness themselves.

The Gay Community

The effects of bereavement and its dynamics cannot be well understood outside the social context within which death occurs. By social context, here the gay community is referred to. Though gay men are members of and take part in the wider societies to which they belong, they have also developed a subculture with a separate ethos. The gay community can be thought of as the overlapping informal social networks of self-identified gay men. While lesbian women are an important and integral part of what is generally regarded as the organized gay community, the extent to which they have been affected by the epidemic and are part of gay men's social networks is not known. It is known, however, that gay men cluster not only in cities, but in neighborhoods or zones of cities, often creating what can be considered gay ghettos (Levine 1989). Frequently they share their homes, vacations and holidays, and patronize business and seek the services of other gay men; many pursue careers and occupations where their co-workers, partners or clients are gay. In addition, gay men frequently remain friends with sex partners and former lovers (domestic partners). In fact, in New York City the typical gay man's primary social network is composed predominantly (60%) of other gay men. This subculture includes among other things a gay sensibility and a liberal political ideology. In part this subculture came about as a result of the lesbian and gay liberation movement of the 1960s and early 1970s (D'Emilio 1983).

Prior to this period homosexuals and their sexual behaviors were considered by the larger society as not only immoral, but illegal and sick. During the period known as gay liberation some of the stigma surrounding homosexuality was alleviated. Gay people protested against discrimination and worked toward changing both antiquated laws prohibiting sodomy, and the medical profession's diagnostic criteria which deemed those who were erotically attracted to members of the same sex as suffering from a psychiatric disorder (Bayer 1981). Gay men became more visible, and they began to assert more positive identity and a more typical (if not exaggerated) masculinity (Marotta 1981). These factors, higher visibility, gay pride and high concentration in cities, brought about institutions and businesses catering for and contributing to the pursuit and expression of previously repressed or covert sexuality (National Research Council 1993). For example, in the pre-AIDS period the majority of New York City gay men between the ages of 30 and 45 participated in a life-style including reciprocal sexual activity with multiple partners (Martin 1987). A large part of this activity took place in sex and dance clubs, public baths and at orgiastic parties in homes. Much of this uninhibited sexual activity occurred in conjunction with the widespread use of an assortment of recreational drugs including alcohol (Martin, Dean, Garcia and Hall 1989).

Sexually transmitted diseases became rampant throughout the gay community. Specialists (both public clinics and private doctors) who treated the prevalent diseases were part of the milieu of gay men. The diseases were tolerated because most were manageable. However, gay men and their physicians were becoming alarmed at the frequency with which these diseases occurred, their increasing chronicity and intractability, and the detrimental effects of the potent medications that were commonly prescribed to alleviate these medical problems. It was within this context that AIDS – then considered a rare and exotic disease – appeared. Because it was first detected in homosexual men it was initially referred to as gay-related immune disorder (GRID). The new disease posed intriguing medical mysteries to which many scientists turned their attention and began to devote their lives (Leibowitch 1985). Gay men living in urban areas were motivated to take part in studies that would elucidate the disease process, help prevent it, hopefully find a cure for those already infected, and to understand its psychosocial consequences. Much of what we now know about AIDS is based on studies of such highly motivated men.

STUDY OF NEW YORK'S GAY COMMUNITY

In 1984 we started a longitudinal, prospective study of the impact of the AIDS epidemic on the health and behavior of New York City gay/bisexual men. We collected data in private, face-to-face interviews held in men's homes using a structured protocol (Martin and Dean 1985–1991) covering a wide range of physical and mental health domains. The study involves 1025 adult gay men whose primary residence was New York City and who had not been diagnosed with AIDS at the time of enrolment. It includes an original cohort and sensitization sample of 851 men aged 18–75 years when enrolled in 1985 and a second cohort of 174 young gay men aged 18–24 when enrolled in 1990. Although the study was initiated as one of 'healthy men' *at risk* for AIDS, it has become one of men who are HIV-seropositive – both asymptomatic and sick with AIDS – and men who are HIV-negative. By 1991 a cumulative total of 138 of the 851 men from the original group had been diagnosed with AIDS, of whom 112 had died.

Sample

No sampling frame exists for enumerating persons according to sexual practices or sexual orientation and therefore we could not draw a random sample of gay men. This is a problem that most researchers studying gay men have faced (Harry 1986). Our solution was to assemble a diverse sample of self-identified gay men from a wide range of sources. We used a variety of methods including (1) a two-stage random sampling (Kish 1965) of members of over 100 gay organizations; (2) 'targeted' or 'applied' sampling methods (Sudman and Kalton 1986) to broaden the scope of the sampling base and (3) 'snowball' (chain referral) sampling (Biernacki and Waldorf 1981) from the social networks of men who completed earlier interviews.

A complete description of our sampling methods is found elsewhere (Martin and Dean 1990, 1993b). It is important to note here that these sampling methods resulted in a broad cross-section of the adult male homosexual community living throughout New York City's five boroughs in 1985. A comparison of the characteristics of the original sample with two gay samples randomly drawn in San Francisco suggests that our study group is as representative of the gay population in New York City as the San Francisco samples were representative of that city's gay population; further, our sample is probably superior to samples of gay men where no efforts were made to draw the study group from diverse channels. HIV infection was neither an exclusion nor an inclusion criterion, but men who had been diagnosed with AIDS by a physician at enrolment were not eligible for the study. The original cohort consisted primarily of well educated men, mean age 36 years, median annual income $25 000. Despite intensive recruitment efforts, only 13% were from ethnic minorities. In all, 42% were coupled with a lover, and 13% were military veterans.

Measures

A full description of study measures used in all seven years, including scale construction, reliability and sources, is available elsewhere. For our bereavement measures we adapted a method for eliciting a social network devised by Phillips and Fischer (1981). We have described these procedures in detail elsewhere (Dean, Hall and Martin 1988; Martin and Dean 1989). Briefly, names were elicited of all the people the respondent knew who had died of AIDS in the 12 months before the interview. We then asked a series of 13 questions about each individual named. In the work presented here we have classified men as AIDS-bereaved if, based on these questions, they have lost either a close friend or a lover to AIDS during the past year. Those who reported no losses during the year, or whose losses were limited to friends and/or acquaintances, were classified as non-bereaved.

Epidemiology of Bereavement

The annual non-cumulative rates of AIDS bereavement in survivors who were willing to be interviewed in all seven years ($n=439$) showed that the experience of AIDS bereavement is ubiquitous in the gay community (Dean 1995). Nearly three-quarters (73%) of the men have experienced at least one major loss. Moreover, the annual rates are not decreasing but increasing, with an incidence averaging 15% in 1985 and 1986, 21% in 1987 and 1988, and 28% in the last two years of the study. Middle-aged men are more likely than either the youngest or oldest to have suffered AIDS bereavement.

In an earlier paper (Martin and Dean 1989) we showed that the AIDS-related deaths and illnesses that occurred early in the epidemic (i.e. up to the end of 1985) were not randomly distributed through New York's gay population. The men who died and the men who mourned them were both clustered in segments of the community who were socially and sexually connected, and the majority were between the ages of 25 and 44. Thus, the bereaved tended not only to be those who were most integrated into the gay community in the beginning of the 1980s but also those most likely to be HIV-positive and to report clinical symptoms of AIDS. Bereaved men were much more sexually active in the year prior to the outbreak of the AIDS epidemic (1980–1981) than men who were not bereaved. Seven years later the pattern holds, although the men have aged, and the experiences of bereavement are more likely to be multiple (more than one annually) and chronic (occurring in consecutive years) rather than single as in the earlier time period.

Psychological Impact of Loss

Our analyses show (Martin 1988; Martin and Dean 1993b) that AIDS-related bereavement early in the epidemic led to distress that is both similar to and different from distress reported in the bereavement literature on heterosexual or general populations (Stroebe and Stroebe 1987). Bereaved gay men, when compared with non-bereaved gay men, were more depressed, considered suicide more frequently, and tended to use or initiate more frequent help from medical, psychological and spiritual professions. Other evidence, however, suggests that gay men also respond to AIDS-related bereavement in unique ways. While they reported elevated levels of anxiety, consistent with the bereavement literature, anxiety among bereaved gay men is highly specific. This anxiety is not a generalized reaction or phobia but rather a disturbing AIDS-specific anxiety (i.e. traumatic stress response symptoms) coupled with a sense of personal vulnerability to developing the disease. As in other samples, bereaved gay men appear vulnerable to increased substance use. But, again, the particular types of substances used by gay men (which include barbiturates, amphetamines and cocaine) are different from those substances (i.e. alcohol and tobacco) which are more often used by other bereaved groups (Clayton 1979; Blankfield 1983).

This study also revealed that multiple and chronic losses lead to levels of AIDS-specific anxiety and subjective sense of threat that go beyond levels associated with a single loss or a loss confined to a remote time period (Martin 1988). To test two competing hypotheses – one drawn from a simple additive model of the effects of stress on well-being often used in theories of grief and loss (see Stroebe and Stroebe 1987) and the other from an adaptation model of repeated experience of stressors (Dubos 1965) – our original cohort was divided into four groups: those who had never been bereaved of a lover or a close friend, those bereaved once, those bereaved twice, and those bereaved three or more times. We found a direct relationship between bereavement episodes and the experience of traumatic stress response symptoms indicative of anxiety, and demoralization, as well as sleep disturbance symptoms, indicating depression. There was a clear lack of relationship between bereavement and problems due to drinking and many forms of drug use, neither of which increased as a function of bereavement. None the less, as the number of bereavements increased, the frequency of using sedatives and recreational drugs other than marijuana or alcohol increased. These results held after adjusting for demographic and health status variables.

There was also a relationship between the number of AIDS-related bereavements and the number of annual consultations with medical specialists: non-bereaved respondents averaged four physician visits per year, while respondents reporting three or more bereavements averaged five physician visits, but there was no clear association between bereavement and the annual number of psychological visits. While the average value is indeed elevated for respondents reporting three or more losses, there is no evidence of average increases in initiating or increasing physician visits associated with one or two bereavements. Measured as a behavioral response to concern over AIDS, however, the relationship between bereavement and initiating or increasing psychological service use appears stronger. Thus 16% of the men who experienced one bereavement had increased or initiated mental health service use, compared with 4% of those who had not been bereaved. This four-fold difference increases to a five-fold difference (20%) among men who experienced three or more bereavements. Of the four measures of help-seeking, only the indicator of initiating or increasing the use of psychological services was significantly related to the frequency of bereavement, after statistically adjusting for demographic and health status factors.

Overall, these findings support a simple additive hypothesis regarding bereavement and signs of distress, namely, as the frequency of loss increases, the frequency of specific psychological symptoms and psychological help-seeking also increases. The data through 1985 did not suggest that adaptation to loss was occurring. At that time we saw no significant decline in symptoms of distress among those who experienced two or more losses.

Resistance and Vulnerability to Loss

As we repeated these measures over time (parelleling the advancing AIDS epidemic), and as we extended the time period over which the effects of bereavement were considered, differences began to emerge between indicators of different types of distress symptoms (Martin and Dean 1993a). For example, scores on the demoralization scale, which includes symptoms commonly found in depression such as negative affect, hopelessness, trouble thinking and low self-esteem, were strongly related to bereavement early in the epidemic; this association diminished over time from 1986 to 1991 (with the exception of 1989 when the association between bereavement and demoralization re-emerged). This pattern of cross-sectional associations is distinctly different from that found for our measure of traumatic stress response: at each time point, from 1985 to 1991, we found a strong and significant relationship between the measures of traumatic stress and bereavement.

During the first five years of the epidemic the cause of AIDS was unknown, its next targets were unknown, and a sense of undifferentiated vulnerability prevailed in urban gay communities. This ambiguity heightened public stigma surrounding AIDS. Such fears and stigma led to increased feelings of social isolation among those with afflicted loved ones. With the exception of the fatality rate for those infected with HIV, the situation has changed dramatically since 1985: the cause of AIDS is known; who will develop AIDS can be known with near certainty; and ways to avoid becoming infected with HIV have been extensively publicized. Although AIDS is still a stigmatized disease and prejudice toward homosexuals exists at a high level (Dean, Wu and Martin 1992), supportive resources for those involved with people with AIDS have grown enormously.

Bereavement and psychological distress are both influenced by many factors. Our work demonstrates that those who are caretakers of people with AIDS and who themselves lack emotional and concrete social support suffer more intense and prolonged grief reactions following the death than do caretakers reporting the presence of reliable support (Lennon, Martin and Dean 1990). We have also shown that being an integrated member of New York's gay community puts one at high risk of being AIDS-bereaved, and that bereavement leads to AIDS activism, including assuming leadership positions in gay organizations and taking care of other sick and bereaved men. Such activism puts one at risk of suffering even more losses (Dean, Hall and Martin 1988).

The changing social context (including the increased willingness of men to seek knowledge of their HIV status) has led to changes in the gay community. The men in this study learned their HIV status only very gradually. The cumulative rate increased as follows: 7% in 1985, 47% in 1988, 85% in 1991 (Dean 1995). Such changes have implications concerning AIDS-related deaths of loved ones. Specifically, we predicted that gay men who knew or believed themselves to be infected with HIV would experience more intense distress because of AIDS-related bereavement compared with men who knew or believed that they were not infected. The basis for this hypothesis was that there would be less room for protective denial (Lazarus 1981) regarding their own fate: men observing the fatal illness of a close friend or lover know that the chances are extremely high that they will be similarly afflicted in a short time period. The salience of bereavement caused by AIDS is thus heightened among this group. By contrast, knowing or believing that one is free of HIV infection provides protective assurance that AIDS-related deaths do not necessarily presage one's own fate. Such knowledge may reduce the salience of negative events such as AIDS-related deaths, rendering them less psychologically distressing. This rationale led us to call this question the 'salience hypothesis'.

Discussion and Implications

These results indicate an historical effect in which the psychological impact of loss is diminishing among gay men who survived the first 10 years of the AIDS epidemic (Martin and Dean 1993a). The strength of the contemporaneous effects of loss (i.e. loss in the prior 12 months) grew progressively smaller each year. In addition, the mental health effects of AIDS-related losses are of a shorter duration in more recent years. In our earlier work we concluded that losses occurring as far back as 1980 contributed to distress levels as much as five years later. On the basis of these later analyses we showed that losses occurring two years before the 1986 and 1987 interviews continued to show significant associations with distress. There were no such two-year effects after 1987. Thus, our findings suggest that both the occurrence and duration of bereavement effects are diminishing with time.

There are several explanations for these diminishing bereavement effects that are consistent with our other findings regarding AIDS and HIV status. Knowing one is HIV-positive or having symptoms of AIDS represents the strongest, most consistent correlate of psychological distress we have found to date. It is reasonable to posit that concern over one's own health status is replacing AIDS losses as the primary determinant of psychological distress among gay men. Our hypothesis that bereavement would have different and stronger effects on the distress levels of AIDS-bereaved HIV-positive men compared with AIDS-bereaved HIV-negative men, was based on the idea that bereavement for the former group would be more salient and thus more distressing because it reminded them of their impending fate.

Another explanation for the diminishing intensity and duration of bereavement effects may lie in the changing characteristics of the cohort. In most cases attrition from this study has been due to AIDS-related illness or death. Thus, the cohort is becoming progressively more homogeneous with respect to being AIDS–HIV-negative. As respondents learn that they are HIV-negative a potent stressor is removed. Bereavement that in previous years was distressing has become less so over time for the men classified as HIV-negative. How HIV-negative men have endured deserves further examination. In future studies of this sample we will explore the mediating roles of personality, social networks and coping strategies such as AIDS activism and volunteering.

Men who are HIV-positive (both those who are bereaved and those who are not) have experienced high levels of distress in all years of the study. More work to elucidate the relationship between psychosocial processes and the course of HIV infection is needed. Although some investigators have not found a relationship between depression and CD4 counts (e.g. Rabkin et al 1991; Perry et al 1992) others have found immune change coincident with bereavement (Burack et al 1993; Kemeny et al 1994). Though the evidence is still limited there is reason to suspect that psychological processes could be associated with immune changes relevant to HIV progression.

Our studies make clear the importance of both the historical and social context in understanding bereavement reactions. In interpreting these findings it should be kept in mind that the relationships we detected occurred among gay men living in an AIDS epicenter and in close contact with AIDS through their community. The distress levels and coping styles of family members, heterosexual friends and neighbors may be very different. In addition, these results cannot be generalized to AIDS-bereaved homosexual men who live far from cities or those who do not identify with a gay community. However, our results test a number of theoretical constructs regarding stress and loss and thus add to the bereavement literature.

ACKNOWLEDGEMENTS

The research described in this chapter and preparation of the chapter were supported by grants from the National Institute of Mental Health MH39557, The Aaron Diamond Foundation, and The New York Community Trust.

REFERENCES

Altman D (1986) *AIDS in the Mind of America: The Social, Political and Psychological Impact of a New Epidemic* Garden City, NY: Anchor Press

Bayer R (1981) *Homosexuality and American Psychiatry: The Politic of Diagnosis* New York: Basic Books

Biernacki P and Waldorf D (1981) Snowball sampling: Problems and techniques of chain referral sampling *Sociol Methods* 10: 141–63

Blankfield A (1983) Grief and alcohol *Am J Drug Alcohol Abuse* 9: 435–46

Burack JH, Barrett DC, Stall RD et al (1993) Depressive symptoms and CD4 lymphocyte decline among HIV-infected men *J Am Med Assoc* 270 (21): 2568–73

Centers for Disease Control (1992) 1993 Revised Classification System for HIV infection and expanded surveillance case definition for AIDS among adolescents and adults. US Department of Health and Human Services *Morbidity and Morality Weekly Report* 41: No. RR–17

Centers for Disease Control (1993) *HIV/AIDS Surveillance Report* Atlanta: Centers for Disease Control

Curran JW, Morgan WM, Hardy AM et al (1985) The epidemiology of AIDS: Current status and future prospects *Science* **229**: 1352–7

Dean L (1995) Psychosocial stressors in a panel of New York City gay men during the AIDS epidemic: 1985–1991. In GM Herek & B Green (eds) *AIDS, Identity and Community* Newbury Park CA: Sage

Dean L, Hall WE & Martin JL (1988) Chronic and intermittent AIDS-related bereavement in a panel of homosexual men in New York City *J Palliat Care* **4**: 54–7

Dean L, Wu S & Martin JL (1992) Trends in violence and discrimination against gay men in New York City, 1984 to 1990. In GM Herek & KT Berrill (eds) *Hate Crimes: Confronting Violence against Lesbians and Gay Men* Newbury Park CA: Sage pp 46–64

D'Emilio J (1983) *Sexual Politics, Sexual Communities: The Making of a Homosexual Minority in the United States, 1940–1970* Chicago: The University of Chicago Press

Dubos R (1965) *Man Adapting* New Haven CT: Yale University Press

Folkman S (1993) Psychosocial effects of HIV infection In L Goldberger & S Breznitz (eds) *Handbook of Stress: Theoretical and Clinical Aspects* 2nd edn New York: Free Press pp 658–81

Harry J (1986) Sampling gay men *J Sex Res* **22**: 21–34

Herek GM (1991) Stigma, prejudice, and violence against gay men. In J Gonsiorek & J Weinrich (eds) *Homosexuality: Research Implications for Public Policy* Newbury Park CA: Sage pp 60–80

Kemeny M, Weiner H, Taylor SE & Schneider S (1994) Repeated bereavement, depressed mood, and immune parameters in HIV seropositive and seronegative gay men *Health Psychol* **13** (1): 14–24

Kish L (1965) *Survey Sampling* New York: Wiley

Lazarus RS (1981) The costs and benefits of denial. In BS Dohrenwend & BP Dohrenwend (eds) *Stressful Life Events and Their Contexts* New York: Prodist pp 131–56

Leibowitch J (1985) *A Strange Virus of Unknown Origin* New York: Random House

Lennon MC, Martin JL & Dean L (1990) The influence of social support on AIDS-related grief reaction among gay men *Soc Sci Med* **31**: 477–84

Levine MP (1989) Gay ghetto *J Homosex* **4**: 363–77

Lopata HZ (1979) *Women as Widows: Support Systems* New York: Elsevier

Lyketsos CG, Hoover DR, Guccione M et al (1990) Depressive symptoms as predictors of medical outcomes in HIV infection *J Am Med Assoc* **270**: (21) 2563–7

Marotta T (1981) *The Politics of Homosexuality* Boston: Houghton Mifflin

Martin JL (1987) The impact of AIDS on gay male sexual behavior patterns in New York City *Am J Public Health* **77**: 580–1

Martin JL (1988) Psychological consequences of AIDS-related bereavement among gay men *J Consult Clin Psychol* **56**: 856–62

Martin JL & Dean L (1985–1991) *The Impact of AIDS on Gay Men: A Research Instrument 1985–1991* (unpublished interview schedule; available from author)

Martin JL & Dean L (1989) Risk factors for AIDS-related bereavement in a cohort of homosexual men in New York City. In B Cooper & T Helgason (eds) *Epidemiology and the Prevention of Mental Disorders* London: Routledge pp 170–84

Martin JL & Dean L (1990) Development of a community sample of gay men for an epidemiologic study of AIDS *Am Behavioral Sci* **33**: 546–61 Reprinted in CM Renzetti and RM Lee (eds) (1993) *Researching Sensitive Topics* Newbury Park: Sage pp 82–99

Martin JL & Dean L (1993a) The effects of AIDS-related bereavement and HIV-related illness on psychological distress among gay men: A seven-year longitudinal study, *J Consult Clin Psychol* **61**: 94–103

Martin JL & Dean L (1993b) Bereavement following death from AIDS: Unique problems, reactions, and special needs. In MS Stroebe W Stroebe & RO Hansson (eds) *Bereavement: A Sourcebook of Research and Intervention* Cambridge: Cambridge University Press pp 317–30

Martin JL, Dean L, Garcia M & Hall W (1989) The impact of AIDS on a gay community: Changes in sexual behavior, substance use, and mental health *Am J Community Psychol* **17**: 269–93

National Research Council (1993) *The Social Impact of AIDS in the United States* Washington DC: National Academy Press

New York City Department of Health, Office of AIDS Surveillance (1993a) *AIDS Surveillance Update 1993*

New York City Department of Health, Office of AIDS Surveillance (1993b) Personal communication, August 1993

Nuland S (1994) *How We Die* New York: Alfred A. Knopf

Parkes CM Weiss RS (1983) *Recovery from Bereavement* New York: Basic Books

Perry S, Fishman B, Jacobsberg L & Frances A (1992) Relationships over 1 year between lymphocyte subsets and psychosocial variables among adults with infection by Human Immunodeficiency Virus *Arch Gen Psych* **49**: 396–401

Phillips SL & Fischer CS (1981) Measuring social support networks in general populations. In BS Dohrenwend & BP Dohrenwend (eds) *Stressful Life Events and Their Contexts* New York: Prodis pp 223–33

Rabkin JG, Williams JB, Goetz R et al (1991) Depression, distress, lymphocyte subsets and human immunodeficiency virus symptoms on two occasions in HIV-positive homosexual men *Arch Gen Psych* **48**: 111–19

Rabkin JG, Williams JBW, Neugebauer R et al (1991) Maintenance of hope in HIV-spectrum homosexual men *Am J Psychiatry* **147**: 1322–6

Shilts R (1987) *And the Band Played On: Politics, People and the AIDS Epidemic* New York: St Martin's Press

Sontag S (1989) *AIDS and Its Metaphors* New York: Farrar Straus and Giroux

Stevens CE, Taylor PE, Zang EA et al (1986) Human T-cell lymphotropic virus type III infection in a cohort of homosexual men in New York City *JAMA* **265**: 2267–72

Stroebe W & Stroebe MS (1987) *Bereavement and Health: The Psychological Consequences of Partner Loss* Cambridge: Cambridge University Press

Sudman S & Kalton G (1986) New developments in the sampling of special populations *Ann Rev Sociol* **12**: 401–29

CHAPTER 3

Suicide in Patients with HIV Infection and AIDS

Kathryn Pugh

The Maudsley Hospital, London, UK

Physical illnesses, particularly those that are life threatening, are associated with increased suicide risk. This is especially the case when patients experience neurological symptoms, including epilepsy and confusional states; these are very common in those with HIV infection, occurring in over 50% of patients.

It would also appear that in general the population in urban environments in the developed world that is particularly affected by HIV infection, is also more vulnerable to emotional difficulties prior to infection; over 30% are likely to have had psychiatric intervention in the past (Atkinson et al 1988; Riccio et al 1993; Pugh et al 1994), and 23% have made past suicide attempts, 17% of these being repeated (Pugh et al 1995).

It is therefore likely that suicide will be a greater risk in patients with AIDS compared with the general population. Up to 45% of patients attending a central London AIDS clinic are psychiatric 'cases' when at this disease stage, the main diagnosis being depression (Pugh et al 1995).

This chapter will provide a brief overview of suicidal behaviour and then consider its particular relation to people with HIV infection and AIDS, with specific reference to the ethical and clinical issues.

There is a close relationship between completed suicide and attempted suicide which relates directly to notions of deliberate self-harm and suicide in the general population.

EPIDEMIOLOGY OF DELIBERATE SELF-HARM

There was a massive increase in attempted suicide in the 1960s and early 1970s (Alderson 1974), especially in self-poisoning. This was followed

Grief and AIDS. Edited by L. Sherr.
©1995 John Wiley & Sons Ltd.

by a decline in rates in the late 1970s and early 1980s (Brewer and Farmer 1985; Platt et al 1988). This decline has halted and may have reversed (Hawton and Fagg 1992) and calculations based on rates in Oxford suggest that there are at least 100 000 hospital referrals per year in England and Wales because of suicide attempts (Hawton and Fagg 1992) while other episodes do not come to medical attention (Kennedy and Kreitman 1973). Attempted suicide is more common in women and in young people, with two-thirds of cases occurring in those under 35 years of age.

EPIDEMIOLOGY OF SUICIDE

Suicide accounts for 1% of deaths annually in the UK. Suicides are frequently recorded as undetermined, so that the figure is probably higher, especially in a population where death is expected from natural causes (Farmer and O'Donnell 1993). Suicides are more common in social classes I and V and occur most frequently in April, May and June. There is an association with particular personality traits and with early life experiences such as a history of bereavement in childhood.

Men outnumber women by 3:1 in terms of completed suicide, and suicide is more common in older than in younger men. However, there has recently been a major change in suicide patterns in young men, in whom rates have increased (Hawton 1992). The rate of suicide has risen by 78% in young men (aged 15–24 years) from 1980 to 1990 (Office of Population Censuses and Surveys 1982, 1991). Suicide is now the second commonest cause of death in young men aged 15–34 years and suicide among young people now accounts for 13% of all suicides. It is notable that rates of death by undetermined causes have risen to a similar extent (Holding and Barraclough 1978). A hypothesis for the increase in suicides in young men is that increasing numbers are remaining single or becoming divorced (suicide rates for men are in the following order: divorced > widowed > single > married). This change is enough to explain about half of the increase between the early 1970s and late 1980s (Charlton et al 1993). This cohort of men have also been affected by high unemployment, well established as associated with suicide (Platt 1984; Smith 1985) as well as with living alone (the important feature being social isolation), increasing risk of imprisonment and the misuse of alcohol and drugs.

Suicide in Persons with Physical Illness

The suicides of young men with HIV infection and AIDS need to be seen in this context, although their experience is also unique to a devastating fatal illness that affects some populations in epidemic proportions.

Physical illness (especially when associated with pain, disability, and a terminal prognosis) is associated with an increased risk of suicide. In studies of patients with cancer the relative risk of suicide is 1.3- to 2-fold that of matched populations (Loutivuon and Hakama 1979; Fox et al 1982; Allebeck and Bolund 1991). A recent history of physical illness is present in a number of people who commit suicide (Barraclough et al 1974; Whitlock 1986; Duggan et al 1991). Physical illness can lead to psychiatric morbidity, especially depression, which in cancer patients, for example, correlates with the progression of the cancer, the level of physical and social support and the number and quality of the frequent losses associated with the cancer (Holland 1978; Pettingale et al 1988).

When illness is associated with neurological complications, for example epilepsy, confusional states, parasthaesia and partial paralysis, the risk of suicide is even greater. In this manner a patient with advanced HIV disease is comparable to an elderly patient, and suicide in the elderly population is the highest, with rates 43% higher than overall population rates.

The phenomenon of underdetection of unnatural deaths is also similar in the elderly population, where suicide may be systematically underdetected (Farmer and O'Donnell 1992). There may be similar underdetection for certain suicide methods. After reviewing 15 000 medicolegal autopsies that had been held for technical reasons, not because the death was considered unnatural, Patel (1974) found 764 elderly people with sufficient poison in their stomach to account for the death.

Previous Histories of Suicidal Behaviour and Completed Suicide

Those who have attempted suicide once represent a 27-fold greater risk of subsequent suicide than the general population (Hawton and Fagg 1988). In a 10-year follow-up of the suicide rate of those persons admitted to a medical ward with self-harm, it was found to be 30 times that expected in the general population (Nordentoft 1993). In the year following the first attempt 1% kill themselves; this is 100 times the rate expected for the general population. The highest risk is in the first 3 years and especially the first 6 months following a suicide act.

In this group the established risk factors for completed suicide are: male sex, social class V, unemployment, repeated deliberate self-harm, substance abuse and a previous psychiatric admission.

Suicide in Relation to Psychiatric Illness

In representative samples of suicide examined using the 'psychological autopsy' method, which consists of interviewing relatives and friends of the deceased as well as scrutinizing the medical records, over 90% have been judged to have some form of psychiatric illness (Barraclough et al 1974; Newson-Smith and Hisch 1979; Urwin and Gibbons 1979). So-called 'rational suicide' is rare in this culture.

Depression is the most frequently specified disorder (47–70%), followed by alcohol dependence (15–27%) and schizophrenia (2–12%) (Robins et al 1959; Dorpat and Ripley 1960; Barraclough et al 1974). The life-time risk of suicide in depression is 15% and in schizophrenia is 10% (Miles 1977) and the life-time risk of suicide in alcohol addiction is 3.4% (Murphy and Wetzer 1990) and is increased in persons with drug addiction. A family history of affective disorder, alcoholism or suicide is also relevant.

PSYCHIATRIC MORBIDITY IN PATIENTS WITH HIV INFECTION AND AIDS

In giving advice to psychiatrists managing patients with HIV (Catalan 1990a) the presence of psychosocial and neuropsychiatric problems is stressed, with a need for careful history taking, not assuming that if a person has HIV disease then the psychiatric illness is related to it, the likelihood being that other factors are predisposing to psychiatric presentation.

With the onset of the AIDS pandemic, considerable attention has been paid to the investigation of the neuropsychiatric aspects (Maj 1990) and psychological impact of HIV infection (Catalan 1990b; Miller and Riccio 1990). The aim of much of the psychological research to date has been to clarify the course of psychological adjustment to the diagnosis and disease progression (Perry et al 1990) and to identify predictors of psychiatric morbidity (Williams et al 1991). Some studies, particularly those that include those with advanced disease, have reported elevated psychiatric morbidity in HIV-seropositive gay or bisexual men (for example, Catalan et al 1992; Pugh 1995) while other studies, particularly those which exclude men with advanced disease, have not found differences associated with HIV serostatus (for example, Atkinson et al 1988; Williams et al 1991; Riccio et al 1993; Pugh et al 1994). It has been suggested that the failure to find differences in psychiatric morbidity associated with HIV status may be because control groups typically consist of HIV-seronegative gay/bisexual men who may themselves suffer significant psychological distress (Ostrow et al 1989; Ostrow, Joseph and Kessler 1989). Several studies conducted before HIV disease was widespread reported a high prevalence of mood abnormalities, and alcohol and drug use by men attending STD clinics, including gay/bisexual men at risk of HIV infection (Pedder and Goldberg 1970; Mayou 1975; Catalan et al 1981; Catalan, Day and Gallway 1988). The implications of these findings are that psychiatric morbidity precedes HIV diagnosis in the majority of patients rather than being a consequence of HIV infection (Atkinson et al 1988; Williams et al 1991) but that advanced HIV disease is an additional factor in increasing psychiatric morbidity (Catalan et al 1992; Pugh et al 1995).

A history of psychiatric illness is the most reliable single predictor of psychiatric morbidity at one-year follow-up of gay/bisexual men recruited from a central London genitourinary medicine clinic who had early HIV disease (CDC II/III) (Pugh et al 1994). Other factors that were associated included young age and illicit drug use, while a belief in the ability of medical professionals to control illness (Locus of Control – Powerful Others) was a protective factor.

A continuation of the same study, including patients with advanced disease, found that 45% of patients with AIDS reached 'caseness' on a standardized psychiatric interview and that this was related not only to more advanced disease stage but more significantly to life experiences in the preceding 6 months (such as death and illness of close friends) and also coping strategies with denial, mental and behavioural disengagement and increased use of drugs and alcohol being associated with psychiatric morbidity (Pugh et al 1995).

Suicidal Intentions in Response to HIV-positive Serostatus

Early studies in New York suggested raised anxiety with suicidal thoughts at the time of HIV testing, which dropped 10 weeks later regardless of subsequent confirmation of serostatus (Perry et al 1990). Similar results were found in London where anxiety at testing was shown to have dropped by one-year follow-up (Pugh et al 1994). Fourteen (25%) recruits were psychiatric 'cases' while awaiting their HIV test results, compared with only three (5%) at one-year follow-up. A similar reduction in psychological distress at follow-up was found with several of the self-report measures of distress. The implication of this reduction in psychological distress is that psychiatric morbidity is related to the stress and uncertainty of HIV testing rather than to serostatus when asymptomatic. On one measure, the Hospital Anxiety and Depression Scale, Subscale Anxiety, HIV serostatus was a significant factor. The reduction in anxiety from baseline to one year was greater for the HIV-positive subjects than for the controls. This is perhaps related to the input of services to individuals with HIV infection, it may reflect a continuing anxiety in the control population remaining at risk of contracting HIV disease (Ostrow, Monjan et al 1989), or alternatively it may be that it represents some form of relief in having a suspected HIV status confirmed.

Around 35% of suicides occur after alcohol has been ingested (The Royal College of Psychiatrists 1979). Alcohol and drug use in the London Clinic population of gay/bisexual men was high at baseline (Pugh et al 1994a), as has been found in other genitourinary medicine settings (Catalan, Day and Gallway 1988), though there is a reduction in alcohol use over time in this cohort regardless of HIV status.

In summary, there is considerable psychiatric morbidity in advanced symptomatic HIV disease while asymptomatic individuals have similar rates to other gay/bisexual men, with the time of HIV testing being anxiety-provoking regardless of serostatus. This corresponds with the findings that suicide increases with disease progression (Marzuk 1991; Mead and Kerkhof 1991; Rajs and Fugelstad 1992; Pugh 1993).

EPIDEMIOLOGY OF SUICIDAL BEHAVIOUR IN PERSONS WITH HIV DISEASE AND AIDS

In a recent estimate of suicide rate in central London in patients registered with AIDS, suicide accounted for 1.7% of deaths in this population (Pugh, O'Donnell and Catalan 1993) compared with around 1% in the general population. In New York a 36-fold increase in relative risk of suicide for men with AIDS, compared with men of the same age group, was reported (Marzuk et al 1988). Caution in interpreting this figure was suggested by the author (Marzuk 1991) as no other factors were controlled for, as in the London data, these being single men in central urban areas and therefore a relatively high-risk group.

Similarly, higher rates of suicide than expected were reported in patients with AIDS elsewhere in the United States (Engelman, Hessol and Lipsom 1988; Kiezer et al 1988). The Department of Forensic Medicine in Stockholm found that the number and proportion of suicides among HIV-positive deaths increased from 1985 to 1990, particularly in the homosexual and bisexual population, and could be related to the duration of infection and to the manifestation of AIDS symptoms (Rajs and Fugelstad 1992). Other authors writing of the situation in Germany, Italy and the Netherlands stressed the lack of reliable data on suicides in the HIV-positive population, due to underreporting of AIDS cases, misclassified deaths and lack of controls in research for other factors independently associated with increased suicide risk (Wedler 1991; Bellini 1991; Mead and Kerkhof 1991).

Epidemiological studies to determine the incidence of suicide are beset with methodological problems (Marzuk 1991). Suicide is a rare event, and so prospective studies are not feasible. There is a high 'natural' morbidity in this patient group and death by 'unnatural' causes is hard to determine. For example, intravenous drug users may have their suicides misclassified as accidental overdoses and deaths in patients with advanced AIDS may be presumed to be the result of infection. If suicide is established it is a further problem to obtain reliable serostatus data and details relevant to suicidal risk for each individual.

The WHO Consultation in Bologna in 1990 made a number of recommendations to improve information on suicide and HIV disease from pathology and forensic departments which included: post-mortem tests for HIV seropositivity on all sudden deaths of uncertain or suspicious cause; the need for neuropathological investigations in HIV patients to investigate possible relationships between neuropathology and suicide as a cause of death; the recording at post-mortem examination on deceased HIV-infected persons of background demographic data, HIV transmission group, drug abuse and alcohol abuse data, past suicide attempts and history of psychiatric treatment; and finally the use of the WHO/CDC criteria for classification of disease development.

There are similar methodological difficulties in the estimation of relative risk of non-fatal suicidal behaviour in patients with HIV disease, as the exact number of persons with HIV infection and the number of persons who harm themselves are not easily available (Catalan 1991). The best predictors of suicidal behaviour in a large cross-sectional Italian study of homosexual men, heterosexual men and intravenous drug users with HIV disease, were previous psychiatric history and past deliberate self-harm. Individuals appeared to be particularly at risk of attempted suicide within the first six months of receiving a diagnosis of HIV and also three years after the diagnosis (Gala et al 1992).

In the Riverside health district of London, verdicts of suicide, undetermined (open) and accidental death were recorded on the death certificate of residents (rather than persons treated) for 1 in 34 (3%) deaths attributable to HIV infection in males aged 15 to 64 years (Aldous et al 1992). The total number of deaths in the Riverside district of patients treated for HIV disease between April 1990 and March 1992 was 363 out of 1901 patients treated. Of these six were known suicides, constituting 0.3% of the total number of patients with known HIV infection treated in the Riverside district between April 1990 and March 1992 and representing 1.7% of the total deaths in this group. This is a minimum estimate, given the possibility that some suicidal deaths may not have come to the researchers' attention (Pugh, O'Donnell and Catalan 1993). The cases in this London study show a number of different points in the aetiology of suicide in patients with HIV disease. The range of time from HIV diagnosis to suicide was six months to six years. Two of the suicides occurred within 16 months of a positive HIV test, and the remaining four occurred between 13 and 25 months after a diagnosis of AIDS. All the patients had a classification of disease of CDCIV (advanced symptomatic HIV disease). A psychiatric history was present in four of the six cases, two preceding the HIV diagnosis, both of whom had made suicide attempts in the past. For the two cases without a psychiatric history, the main motive appeared to be release from a debilitating and fatal illness. In one case the decision had been made a year in advance.

The choice of suicide method was predominantly by jumping (four of six), the remaining two being overdoses. This is an extremely high proportion compared with the general population rate in men of 7% by jumping (OPCS 1991). The method of jumping from a height or under a moving train accounted for two-thirds of the suicides in the London sample (Pugh, O'Donnell and Catalan 1993) and the New York finding (Marzuk 1991), but is not reflected in other findings of 15% and 10% in patients with AIDS (Kiezer et al 1988; Rajs and Fugelstad 1992), and 12% in patients with cancer (Allebeck and Bolund 1991) which approach population norms of 7% in males (OPCS 1991). It may be that there is underdetection of suicides in the HIV population, especially of overdoses, thus leading to a misleadingly high picture of jumping as a method of choice. However, the choice of jumping as a method of suicide may reflect a real difference between suicide in this sample compared with men in the general population and may be related to psychiatric and medical morbidity.

The past history of deliberate self-harm in two of the six suicides, and a past history of psychiatric intervention in four cases of the London sample (Pugh, O'Donnell and Catalan 1993) resembles Marzuk's findings in the 12 suicides that occurred in men with AIDS in New York in 1985, of whom one-third had histories of previous suicide attempts and one-half had a diagnosis of depression in the preceding month (Marzuk et al 1988). One patient in the London sample had seen a psychiatrist within four days of the suicide. This was the case in half of the suicides reported by Marzuk. In their study on attempted suicide in patients with HIV disease the Italian psychiatric team found a previous history of deliberate self-harm and a previous psychiatric history to be the best predictors of suicidal behaviour (Gala et al 1992).

The importance of life events in suicidal behaviour in patients with HIV disease is highlighted in the London sample where suicide was preceded by bankruptcy, death of father (anniversary reaction) and recent refugee status in addition to physical illness events, and these factors have been noted as associated with suicide in epidemiological surveys in the general population (Barraclough and Hughes 1987). HIV-specific events such as HIV diagnosis, AIDS diagnosis and sudden deterioration in health were perhaps triggers for the suicidal behaviour, as is found in the Italian study on attempted suicide (Gala et al 1992). Other writers have proposed a model of cumulative stressors leading to suicide, for example, bereavements, illness in friends and episodes of ill health (Schneider et al 1991a). HIV-seropositive individuals may have a different susceptibility to AIDS-related stressors, such as illness and deaths in friends, than HIV-seronegative individuals, as they anticipate their own illness progression within a relatively concentrated social network of friends with HIV infection (Schneider et al 1991b).

ETHICAL ISSUES

Suicide in persons with AIDS may appear on the surface to be a form of self-administered euthanasia, a 'rational suicide', of little concern to mental health professionals. Persons with a debilitating, painful and fatal illness have the right to die in a dignified and controlled way and this issue of 'living wills' with restriction of medical intervention at the end of life and sufficient effective pain relief must be considered with the issue of suicide. Work in the Netherlands where euthanasia is available suggests that good hospice care has a significant effect in reducing the request for euthanasia.

The ethical issues in the euthanasia debate have attracted attention in the United States and elsewhere (Beckett 1991; Catalan 1991) and may involve mental health professionals who are called upon to assess the mental state of AIDS patients with suicidal ideation.

ASSESSING/MANAGING SUICIDE RISK

The majority of people who kill themselves (Barraclough et al 1974) or who make attempts (Hawton and Blackstock 1976; Bancroft et al 1977) have been in recent contact with doctors, usually GPs and also psychiatrists. This is equally true for HIV patients (Marzuk 1991; Pugh, O'Donnell and Catalan 1993). Despite this opportunity for intervention it is recognized that it is difficult to assess suicide risk (Hawton 1987).

One of the suicides in the London sample occurred on a medical ward. The New York study reported 25% of the cases as occurring during admission (Marzuk et al 1988). This is perhaps inevitable when patients with AIDS spend so much time on medical wards following their diagnosis. The role of the liaison psychiatrist in the setting of a genitourinary medicine clinic and acute medical ward will not only be to assess the mental state of patients but also to support nursing and medical staff in their assessments and management of suicidal patients. It has been established that nurses can effectively assess most self-poisoning patients in a general medical setting provided they have received appropriate training (Catalan et al 1980) and this has been recognized as an important service provision in medical settings dealing with patients with AIDS (Nymathi and van Servellen 1989).

Educational programmes for GPs to detect and treat depression were found to be effective in decreasing the rate of suicide, with these pronounced effects lasting for two years only (Rutz, Knorring and Walinder 1989, 1992). The authors suggest a need for training of GPs to include seminar groups and not written material alone (Michel and Valach 1992).

Although a substantial proportion of people who kill themselves have seen their GPs in the preceding four weeks (in a Bristol study 36%), this is not the case in young persons (under 35) and the reason for this is not clear. Some authors consider that this group are less likely to see it as appropriate to talk to doctors about emotional difficulties and their suicide acts may be more impulsive (Vassilas and Morgan 1993).

Psychological, social and biological factors combine and interact as important contributors in trying to reach an understanding of the suicide act. Knowledge of the suicidal state of mind has been gathered from 500 interviews over a four-year period with patients who were seen within 24 hours of a suicidal act and during psychoanalytic therapy with 20 patients following a suicide act (Campbell and Hale 1991). The suicidal state of mind is described as one of extreme ambivalence where fear of abandonment or engulfment is directed towards the self's body, instead of an external object, and a fantasy is that the body must be killed if the self is to survive. There can be a number of fantasies of the 'surviving self'. One is a 'merging self', where the body is seen as an impediment to the fulfilling of a fantasy of merging with a 'blissful universe'; another is a retaliating, revenging and triumphant self: 'they will be sorry'; a third is self-punishment, dominated by guilt; a fourth, an elimination fantasy: 'kill the body before it kills me'; and the fifth is a 'dicing with death' fantasy which may be especially relevant where sexual behaviour itself may be like playing Russian roulette.

It may be useful to be aware that such fantasies may be operating in someone who presents after a suicide attempt, and an opportunity to discuss these in a therapeutic relationship could enable a change in their state of mind and thus reduce the future risk of suicide.

Morgan (1993) describes patients who commit suicide as falling into two stereotypes; those with 'real depression' or those with 'personality disorder'. What he believes is common to *all* is the presence of alienation.

This alienation is not only in the patient's personal life but becomes re-enacted with health professionals. It is common to find negative attitudes towards patients who subsequently commit suicide. Morgan (1993) poses the following question, that might especially be asked regarding a patient with a fatal illness such as AIDS:

Q Sometimes a person's life situation becomes truly hopeless and impossible to face. In such circumstances should not suicide be regarded as the best solution for that individual?

He also provides a possible response:

A Even simple listening can help alleviate such despair. Many would claim that we should do all we can to prevent the extreme psychological distress of terminal despair.

REFERENCES

Alderson MR (1974) Self-poisoning: what is the future? *Lancet* i: 1040–3

Aldous J, Hickman M, Ellam A et al (1992) Impact of HIV infection in young men in a London health authority *BMJ* **305**: 219–21

Allebeck P & Bolund C (1991) Suicide and suicide attempts in cancer patients *Psychol Med* **21**: 979–84

Atkinson J, Grant I, Kennedy C et al (1988) Prevalence of psychiatric disorders among men infected with human immunodeficiency virus *Arch Gen Psychiatry* **45**: 859–64

Bancroft J, Skrimshire A, Casson J et al (1977) People who deliberately poison or injure themselves: their problems and their contacts with helping agencies *Psychol Med* **7**: 289–303

Barraclough BM, Bunch J, Nelson B & Sainsbury P (1974) A hundred cases of suicide: clinical aspects *Br J Psychiatry* **125**: 355–73

Barraclough B & Hughes J (1987) *Suicide: Clinical and Epidemiological Studies* London: Croom Helm

Beckett A (1991) Ethical issues in the psychiatry of HIV disease *Int Rev Psychiatry* **3**: 417–28

Bellini M (1991) Considering AIDS/HIV infection and suicidality in Italy. In JE Beskow, M Bellini, JG Sampaio Faria & AD Kerkhof (eds) *HIV and AIDS-related Suicidal Behaviour. Report on a WHO Consultation, Bologna, September 22–23, 1990* Bologna: Monduzzi Editore pp 45–54

Brewer C & Farmer R (1985) Self-poisoning in 1984: a prediction that didn't come true *BMJ* **290**: 391

Campbell D & Hale R (1991) Suicidal acts. In J Holmes (ed) *Textbook of Psychotherapy in Psychiatric Practice* London: Churchill Livingstone pp 287–306

Catalan J (1990a) HIV and AIDS-related psychiatric disorder: what can psychiatrists do? In K Hawton & P Cowen (eds) *Dilemmas and Difficulties in the Management of Psychiatric Patients* Oxford: Oxford University Press pp 236–58

Catalan J (1990b) Psychiatric manifestations of HIV disease *Baillières Clin Gastroenterol* **4**: 547–62

Catalan J (1991) Deliberate self-harm in HIV disease. Research into clinical and ethical aspects. In JE Beskow, M Bellini, JG Sampaio Faria & AD Kerkhof (eds) *HIV and AIDS-related Suicidal Behaviour. Report on a WHO Consultation, Bologna, September 22–23, 1990* Bologna: Monduzzi Editore pp 61–8

Catalan J, Day A & Gallway J (1988) Alcohol misuse in patients attending a genitourinary clinic *Alcohol Alcohol* **23**: 421–8

Catalan J, Bradley M, Gallway J & Hawton K (1981) Sexual dysfunction and psychiatric morbidity in patients attending a clinic for sexually transmitted diseases *Br J Psychiatry* **138**: 292–6

Catalan J, Klimes I, Day A et al (1992) The psychosocial impact of HIV infection in gay men: a controlled investigation and factors associated with psychiatric morbidity *Br J Psychiatry* **161**: 774–8

Catalan J, Marsack P, Hawton K et al (1980) Comparison of doctors and nurses in the assessment of deliberate self-poisoning patients *Psychol Med* **10**: 483–91

Charlton J, Kelly S, Dunnell K et al (1993) Suicide deaths in England and Wales: trends in factors associated with suicide deaths *Popul Trends* **71**: 34–42

Dorpat TL & Ripley HS (1960) A study of suicide in the Seattle area *Compr Psychiatry* **1**: 349–59

Duggan CF, Sham P, Lee AS & Murray RM (1991) Can future suicidal behaviour in depressed patients be predicted? *J Affect Disord* **22**: 111–18

Engelman J, Hessol N & Lipsom A (1988) Suicide patterns and AIDS in San Francisco *IV Int Conf AIDS* (Stockholm) Abstr 8597

Farmer R & O'Donnell I (1993) Suicide by poisoning in elderly populations. In K Bohme & H Wedler (eds) *Suicidal Behaviour: The State of the Art* Regensburg: Roderer Verlag

Fox BH, Stanek EJ, Boyd SC & Flanney JT (1982) Suicide rates among cancer patients *Conn J Chronic Dis* **35**: 85–100

Gala C, Pergami A, Catalan J et al (1992) Risk of deliberate self-harm and factors associated with suicidal behaviour among asymptomatic individuals with HIV infection. *Acta Psychiatr Scand* **86**(1): 70–5

Hawton K (1987) Assessment of suicide risk *Br J Psychiatry* **150**: 145–53

Hawton K (1992) By their own hand: suicide is increasing rapidly in young men (Editorial) *BMJ* **304**: 1000

Hawton K & Blackstock E (1976) General practice aspects of self-poisoning and self injury *Psychol Med* **6**: 571–5

Hawton K & Fagg J (1988) Suicide, and other causes of death following attempted suicide *Br J Psychiatry* **152**: 359–66

Hawton K & Fagg J (1992) Trends in deliberate self poisoning and self injury in Oxford, 1976–1990 *BMJ* **304**: 1409–11

Holding TA & Barraclough BM (1978) Undetermined deaths – suicide or accident? *Br J Psychiatry* **133**: 542–9

Holland JC (1978) Psychological aspects of cancer. In JC Holland et al (eds) *Cancer Medicine* 2nd edn Philadelphia: Lea and Febiger

Kennedy P & Kreitman N (1973) An epidemiological survey of parasuicide (attempted suicide) in general practice *Br J Psychiatry* **123**: 23–34

Kiezer K, Green M, Perkins C et al (1988) AIDS and suicide in California *JAMA* **260**: 1881

Loutivuon KA & Hakama M (1979) Risk of suicide among cancer patients *Am J Epidemiol* **109**: 59–65

Maj M (1990) Psychiatric aspects of HIV infection and AIDS *Psychol Med* **20**: 547–63

Marzuk PM (1991) Suicidal behaviour and HIV illnesses *Int Rev Psychiatry* **3**: 367

Marzuk P, Tierney H, Tardiff K et al (1988) Increased risk of suicide in patients with AIDS *JAMA* **259**: 1333–7

Mayou R (1975) Psychological morbidity in a clinic for sexually transmitted disease *Br J Venereal Dis* **51**: 57–60

Mead C & Kerkhof A (1991) Considerations on suicidal behaviour among AIDS and HIV infected patients in the Netherlands. In JE Beskow, M Bellini, JG Sampaio Faria & AD Kerkhof (eds) *HIV and AIDS-related Suicidal Behaviour. Report on a WHO Consultation, Bologna, September 22–23 1990* Bologna: Monduzzi Editore pp 55–60

Michel K & Valach L (1992) Suicide prevention: spreading the gospel to general practitioners *Br J Psychiatry* **160**: 757–60

Miles CP (1977) Conditions predisposing to suicide: a review *J Nerv Ment Dis* **164**: 231–46

Miller D & Riccio M (1990) Editorial review: non-organic psychiatric and psychosocial syndromes associated with HIV-1 infection and disease *AIDS* **4**: 381–8

Morgan HG (1993) *Suicide Prevention: The Assessment and Management of Suicide Risk. A Guide for Health Care Professionals* University of Bristol (unpublished)

Murphy GE & Wetzer RD (1990) The lifetime risk of suicide in alcoholism *Arch Gen Psychiatry* **47**: 383–92

Newson-Smith JG & Hisch S (1979) Psychiatric symptoms in self poisoning patients *Psychol Med* **9**: 493–500

Nordentoft M, Breun L, Munde LK et al (1993) High mortality by natural and unnatural causes *BMJ* **30**(6893): 1637–41

Nymathi A & Van Servellen G (1989) Maladaptive coping in the critically ill population with acquired immunodeficiency syndrome, nursing assessment and treatment *Heart Lung* **18**(2): 113–20

Office of Population Censuses and Surveys (1982) *Mortality Statistics for England and Wales 1980* London: HMSO (DH2 Series No 7)

Office of Population Censuses and Surveys (1991) *Mortality Statistics for England and Wales 1990* London: HMSO (DH2 Series No 17)

Ostrow D, Monjan A, Joseph J et al (1989) HIV related symptoms and psychological functioning in a cohort of homosexual men *Am J Psychiatry* **146**: 737–42

Ostrow D, Joseph J & Kessler R (1989) Disclosure of HIV antibody status: behavioural and mental correlates *AIDS Educ Prev* **146**: 1–11

Patel NS (1974) A study on suicide *Med Sci Law* **14**(2): 129–36

Pedder JR & Goldberg D (1970) A survey by questionnaire of psychiatric disturbance in patients attending a venereal disease clinic *Br J Venereal Dis* **46**: 58–61

Perry S, Jacobsberg L, Fishman B et al (1990) Psychological responses to serological testing for HIV *AIDS* **4**: 145–52

Pettingale KW, Burgess C & Greer A (1988) Psychological response to cancer diagnosis. One constellation with prognostic variables *J Psychosom Res* **32**: 255–61

Platt S (1984) Unemployment and suicidal behaviour – a review of the literature *Soc Sci Med* **19**: 93–115

Platt S, Hawton K, Kreitman N et al (1988) Recent clinical and epidemiological trends in parasuicide in Edinburgh and Oxford: A tale of two cities *Psychol Med* **18**: 405–18

Pugh K, O'Donnell I & Catalan J (1993) Suicide and HIV disease *AIDS Care* **5**: 391–9

Pugh K, Burgess AP, Lovett E et al (1994a) A longitudinal study of the neuropsychiatric consequences of HIV-1 infection in gay men: II – Health and psychological status at baseline and 12 month follow-up *Psychol Med* **24**: 897–904

Pugh K, Catalan J, Lovett E et al (1994b) Factors associated with psychiatric morbidity in men with HIV infection: life experiences, coping strategies and disease stage Submitted

Rajs J & Fugelstad A (1992) Suicide related to immunodeficiency virus infection in Stockholm *Acta Psychiatr Scand* **85**: 234–9

Riccio M, Pugh K, Jadresic D et al (1993) Neuropsychiatric aspects of HIV-1 infection in gay men: controlled investigation of psychiatric, neuropsychological and neurological status *J Psychosom Res* **37**(6): 1–12

Robins E, Murphy GE, Wilkinson R H et al (1959) Some clinical considerations in the prevention of suicide based on a study of 134 successful suicides *Am J Public Health* **49**: 888–99

The Royal College of Psychiatrists (1979) *Alcohol and Alcoholism. The Report of a Special Committee of the Royal College of Psychiatrists* London: Tavistock Press

Rutz W, Knorring L & Walinder J (1989) Frequency of suicide on Gotland after systematic postgraduate education of general practitioners *Acta Psychiatr Scand* **80**: 151–4

Rutz W, Knorring L & Walinder J (1992) Long-term effects of an educational program for general practitioners given by the Swedish Committee for the Prevention and Treatment of Depression *Acta Psychiatr Scand* **85**: 83–8

Schneider SG, Taylor SE, Kernery ME & Hammen C (1991a) AIDS related factors predictive of suicidal ideation of low and high intent among gay and bisexual men *Suicide Life Threat Behav* **21**: 228–313

Schneider SG, Taylor SE, Hammen C et al (1991b) Factors influencing suicide intent in gay and bisexual suicide ideators: differing models for men with and without human immunodeficiency virus *J Pers Soc Psychol* **61**: 776–88

Smith R (1985) 'I couldn't stand it anymore': unemployment and suicide *BMJ* **291**: 1563–6

Urwin P & Gibbons JL (1979) Psychiatric diagnosis in self-poisoning patients *Psychol Med* **9**: 501–7

Vassilas CA & Morgan HM (1993) General Practitioner's contact with victims of suicide *BMJ* **307**: 300–1

Wedler H (1991) Suicidal behaviour in the HIV infected population. The actual situation in the FRG. In JE Beskow, M Bellini, JG Sampaio Faria & AD Kerkhof (eds) *HIV and AIDS-related Suicidal Behaviour. Report on a WHO Consultation, Bologna, September 22–23, 1990* Bologna: Monduzzi Editore pp 41–4

Whitlock FA (1986) Suicide and physical illness. In A Roy (ed) *Suicide* Baltimore: Williams and Wilkins

Williams J, Rabkin J, Remien R et al (1991) Multidisciplinary baseline assessment of homosexual men with and without human immunodeficiency virus infection. II. Standardized clinical assessment of current and lifetime psychopathology *Arch Gen Psychiatry* **48**: 124–30

CHAPTER 4

Psychiatric Problems Associated with Grief

J Catalan

Charing Cross and Westminster Medical School, London, UK

The capacity to become attached to others and to develop emotional bonds is a fundamental characteristic of human beings, and one which is closely related to our ability to survive as a species. The experience of psychological and social distress when faced with threatened or actual loss or separation is an integral part of the same process. Although the neurobiological basis of attachment is not well understood (see Reite and Field (1985) for review), its psychological and social correlates in humans have been described (Parkes 1972; Bowlby 1977a, 1977b).

Grief is a universal human experience but its manifestations are variously influenced by many factors, such as the circumstances of the death, the nature of the relationship between the bereaved and the dead person, the personality and other characteristics of the bereaved, and the social, cultural and interpersonal circumstances of the survivor. The majority of bereaved individuals experience a pattern of psychological distress and social dysfunction which is within the culturally sanctioned range of responses, while a substantial minority suffer more significant and severe disruption of their psychological and social functioning. It is in such cases that the term 'pathological grief' is used (Engel 1961). While there is a risk of medicalizing grief, as in the case of other human experiences like birth and death, it has to be recognized that for some individuals, grief can reach an intensity or duration of such degree that it interferes significantly with the person's life. Furthermore, individuals experiencing pathological grief can benefit from specific psychological and social interventions.

Grief and AIDS. Edited by L. Sherr.
©1995 John Wiley & Sons Ltd.

In this chapter the characteristics of normal and pathological grief, with reference to HIV infection, are reviewed, and the range of specialized psychiatric interventions available considered.

NORMAL GRIEF

Grief as a Process of Adaptation to Loss

The psychological, biological and social consequences of loss and bereavement have been the subject of a variety of descriptive studies (see, for example, Lindemann 1944; Parkes 1972). The impact of loss, threatened or actual, has been conceptualized in several ways, although a common theme to them all is the perception of grief as a process and therefore a changeable phenomenon, rather than as a static event.

Kubler-Ross (1969) thinks of mourning as evolving through a number of 'stages': denial and isolation; anger; bargaining; depression; and acceptance, while stressing that these are not inevitable or fixed in their occurrence. Others like Parkes (1970, 1972) and Bowlby (1980) view grief as involving 'phases': numbness; yearning and anger; disorganization and despair; and reorganization. Worden (1992) uses the concept of 'tasks of mourning': acceptance of the reality of the loss; working through the pain of grief; adjustment to an environment without the deceased person; and emotional relocation of the dead person. It has been argued that the idea of tasks adds a sense of activity and working through on the part of the bereaved and the opportunity to focus on specific aspects of the process to achieve its completion (Worden 1992).

Jacobs (1993) has attempted to provide an account of the features of grief within the model of attachment theory, using the concept of 'dimensions' of grief, interrelated manifestations of mourning which evolve independently over time. Following a period of numbness or unreality, separation pain or distress would emerge (Raphael 1983). Separation distress is regarded as a fundamental feature of grief, being characterized by yearning, preoccupation with the deceased, crying, searching, anger and anxiety. The acute features of separation distress do fade gradually, while the depressive symptoms and manifestations of mourning tend to persist and possibly worsen over time, with sadness, despair, insomnia, lethargy and loss of interest in one's surroundings. The process of recovery and use of adaptive coping responses continues while the other manifestations of grief (sadness, lethargy) are still present. As with other descriptions and formulations of the manifestations of grief, there are unresolved questions about their empirical and theoretical strength.

Factors Associated With the Manifestation of Grief

Not everyone responds to loss in a predictable, standard way, and it is clear that the descriptions of the process of normal grief provide only an idealized model of the process. In practice, a variety of psychological and social factors will contribute to modulate the expression of grief. Worden (1992) has summarized its most important determinants, including: who the person was (partner as opposed to distant relative); the nature of the relationship (its strength, security, ambivalence and conflicts); mode of death (expected, suicidal or in tragic circumstances); past experience of losses; personality of the bereaved; social variables and supports; and the existence of concurrent stresses.

The above factors will influence the way in which grief is manifested, and they will also play a part in the development of pathological grief by contributing to its intensity and features, and to its course over time. HIV infection provides a fertile ground for the development of pathological grief, as other chapters in this volume highlight. The stigma associated with the disease can lead to reduced social supports and rejection by others, fears of contagion may affect partners and relatives, exposure to multiple losses is likely to lead to increased difficulty accepting the reality of the loss and the expression of affect, death of young individuals does increase the sense of waste and sadness, and the painful and disfiguring complications can add to the persistence of disturbing memories for the bereaved. Child death followed by parental death can lead to problems for the surviving children. Often, relatives have been kept in the dark about the disease until rather late in the condition, curtailing the length of time that they can devote to caring for the sick person.

PATHOLOGICAL GRIEF

As in the case of normal grief, there have been many attempts to develop a conceptual understanding of pathological grief (Freud 1917; Deutsch 1937; Lindemann 1944; Bowlby 1980) and also to obtain empirical evidence for its characteristics and course (Parkes 1970; Clayton 1990; Jacobs et al 1989, 1990). In comparison with uncomplicated grief, pathological grief will be characterized by marked differences in its intensity, specific manifestations and evolution over time. While it is not always easy to differentiate normal and abnormal grief, there have been useful attempts to provide operational definitions (see Jacobs 1993). In some cases, grief can lead to clear-cut and well recognized psychiatric syndromes, such as major depression or anxiety disorders, where the bereavement has acted as a precipitant for the psychiatric disorder.

Lazare (1979) has suggested a number of useful clues to identify pathological grief: the person cannot talk about the deceased without experiencing fresh grief; minor events trigger off an intense grief response; loss is often a topic of conversation; reluctance to move the deceased's belongings; the bereaved reports physical symptoms similar to those of the dead person; radical and sudden lifestyle changes following the loss; or the presence of death or illness fears and phobias.

The frequency with which pathological grief occurs will depend to some extent on the criteria used to define it, but a commonly mentioned figure is that quoted by Jacobs (1993), who states that about 20% of bereaved individuals experience pathological grief.

From a practical point of view, pathological grief will be discussed under the following headings: (a) absent or delayed grief; (b) chronic grief; (c) inhibited or distorted grief; (d) severe grief; (e) grief associated with significant psychiatric syndromes.

Absent or Delayed Grief

In this form of pathological grief there is absence or delay of the manifestations of numbness and disbelief, separation distress and subsequent features usually associated with normal grief, for a period of at least two weeks. In some cases, the delay may be a matter of months or even years. Not infrequently, further losses or seemingly less significant experiences of sadness may act as triggers for the onset of obvious grief.

Delay in the process of grieving may be the result of the traumatic nature of the loss, or due to the presence of other pressing difficulties which absorb the attention and emotions of the bereaved person, preventing the usual expression of feelings.

. . . .

A striking example of absent grief was seen by the author in the case of a young man, himself with HIV infection, who had been involved in the 'mercy killing' of his partner who was suffering from advanced HIV infection. After reporting the case to the police, he was tried and given a prison sentence, and when released two years after the death of his partner, he was still unable to acknowledge the loss or to respond emotionally to their former joint surroundings. He did not experience any distress or sadness, but had some insomnia and a marked sense of disorientation and inability to plan for the future. While he remembered clearly the events of the last couple of years, they felt as if someone else had experienced them.

. . . .

Absent or delayed grief should not be confused with the presence of mild manifestations of mourning in someone who has experienced grief prior to the actual loss, as for example in the case of a person nursing and looking after a loved one during terminal illness. The term 'anticipatory grief' (Lindemann 1944) has been used to describe this form of normal grief.

Chronic Grief

In normal grief there is a good deal of variation in the duration of the manifestations of mourning, although it is usually assumed that it is within the first year that most of the distressing features occur. Anniversary reactions are regarded as normal even many years after the loss. In chronic grief there is not only persistence over time in the intensity of thoughts and emotions associated to the deceased, but there is also a subjective sense of not being able to return to normal living and of not having worked through the process of mourning. In the terminology of Worden (1992), the tasks of mourning have not been completed, so that the reality of the loss may not have been accepted, adjustment to an environment without the deceased has not begun to happen, or the dead person has not been emotionally relocated by the bereaved. Preoccupation with the grave, either resulting in avoidance of visits, or very frequent visiting is not uncommon. Sometimes the room and possessions of the deceased are left unchanged, as if waiting for the person to return. The bereaved person's life remains dominated by the deceased, without returning to a normal life and to the exclusion of other relationships. While symptoms of anxiety or depression may be present, they do not usually reach the severity of a clinical psychiatric syndrome.

. . . .

One such case of persistent grief was observed in a man with AIDS whose partner, also with AIDS, died suddenly in his presence from a heart attack. Their relationship had always been difficult, and the survivor blamed his partner for having infected them both with HIV. Anger at his partner's behaviour and guilt for not having prevented his sudden death were prominent and conflicting emotions that persisted for the rest of his life.

. . . .

Inhibited or Distorted Grief

Instead of the usual phases or tasks seen in normal mourning, an erratic pattern of emotional responses and thoughts is present, without a clear evolutionary progress. Complaints of somatic symptoms (headaches, palpitations), anxiety or depression, or behavioural manifestations such as hostility, displaced anger, overidentification with the deceased, may become more prominent than the usual features of grief. As in chronic grief, the person may be aware of not working through the loss.

· ·

Following the death by suicide of a close friend with AIDS, the bereaved person, already HIV symptomatic, developed severe headaches and leg weakness, and severe insomnia. He understood the relationship between his symptoms and the loss, but had greater difficulty recognizing that his many arguments with doctors, social workers and others involved in his own care were related to his feelings that they had let his friend down in some way, leaving the bereaved person as the only one involved in providing support, and thus making him feel responsible for his death.

· ·

Severe Grief

The difference between normal and severe grief is only one of degree, with marked separation distress, crying, yearning, somatic manifestations and perceptual and cognitive disturbances. The severity of the early features of grief may be a predictor of chronic grief.

Grief Associated with Psychiatric Disorders

Whatever the pattern of the grief reaction, some individuals may develop frank psychiatric syndromes in association with the loss. In some cases, the person may have experienced similar problems in response to other undesirable life events, suggesting the presence of vulnerability or predisposition to psychiatric disorders. When grief is associated with significant psychiatric disturbance, it is legitimate to assess and manage the problem taking into account both the precipitant (the loss) and the characteristics of the specific syndrome, so as to provide effective help.

The most frequently seen psychiatric syndromes are post-traumatic stress disorders, depressive disorders and anxiety disorders.

Post-traumatic Stress Disorder (PTSD)

The revised third edition (APA 1987) of the *Diagnostic and Statistical Manual* (DSM–III–R) defines PTSD as the syndrome that occurs following a traumatic event and that includes recurrent and intrusive distressing recollections, dreams or feelings related to the event, persistent avoidance of the above, and symptoms of persistent arousal. While some of its features are not unlike those of normal grief, here they are characterized by their intensity and the traumatic, sudden and often horrific nature of the death.

Depressive Disorders

In the initial stages of grief there are many similarities to major depression. An understandable mood disturbance of this kind can, however, evolve into a major depressive disorder, characterized by the presence of depressed mood, loss of interest in things, loss of pleasure, somatic symptoms such as loss of weight, appetite and early morning waking, feelings of worthlessness and guilt, suicidal ideas, and agitation or psychomotor retardation (Gelder, Gath and Mayou 1989). In major depressive disorders the feelings of worthlessness and guilt tend to be generalized, rather than focused on the deceased. DSM–III–R also lists dysthymia or depressive neurosis amongst the depressive disorders, a condition characterized by less severe symptoms of depression but with a tendency to chronicity, as is often seen in chronic grief. It is important to identify depressive disorders in people who have faced a bereavement, as it may be necessary to consider the use of medication and other psychiatric treatments.

There is an increased risk of suicide behaviour after bereavement, both completed suicide and deliberate self-harm (see Jacobs (1993) for review), and in many such cases major depression is likely to be implicated.

Anxiety Disorders

Anxiety symptoms are common in mourning, in particular in the early stages, but well circumscribed anxiety disorders can develop in association with bereavement, such as generalized anxiety, panic and phobic disorders (Gelder, Gath and Mayou 1989). In some cases anxiety disorders occur in the context of chronic or inhibited grief, but they may require treatment in their own right.

Other Psychiatric Disorders

In vulnerable individuals, bereavement can lead to a wide range of psychiatric syndromes and behavioural problems, grief having acted as trigger for the disorder. Examples will include alcohol- and drug-related problems, antisocial acts, and dissociative and somatoform disorders (Gelder, Gath and Mayou, 1989).

PSYCHIATRIC MANAGEMENT OF GRIEF

Worden (1992) has made a useful distinction between 'grief counselling' – help to facilitate normal, uncomplicated grief – and 'grief therapy' – interventions to help resolve pathological grief. In practice, most people faced with uncomplicated grief do not come near professionals with particular expertise in the field, although they may well come into contact with health and social workers who are in a good position to facilitate or hinder their mourning. Even amongst those experiencing pathological grief, only a minority are likely to receive appropriate specialist care. Many factors contribute to this failure to identify and help those with grief-related problems, amongst them reluctance to regard a private and personal experience of loss as something requiring professional help, and lack of adequately trained professionals.

Facilitating Normal Grief

As described above, mourning is an active process which involves tasks, stages or phases, and the role of facilitating normal grief involves working with the bereaved person to work through and complete this process. Few people experiencing grief will seek professional help, the majority being supported by friends and relatives. Some, however, will come into contact with statutory or independent sources of help. In most instances, the person providing help will take a rather non-interventionist role, encouraging and giving permission for the person to explore and experience feelings and thoughts, rather than prescribing a particular kind of mourning.

While there are different techniques and approaches to grief counselling, in practice there are some shared themes. Worden (1992) has described ten principles to help the bereaved person work through grief:

1 Help to actualize the loss, for example by encouraging description of the death and its circumstances and aftermath.
2 Help to identify and express feelings, in particular anger and guilt, which may be regarded as unacceptable.
3 Help to start living without the dead person, which may involve making decisions and changes without being frozen by the need to guess what the dead person might have done or expected.
4 Help to relocate the dead person emotionally, in particular regarding establishing new relationships.
5 Allow time to grieve, recognizing that the whole process does take time, and giving the bereaved permission to do it at their own pace.
6 Reassure the bereaved about the normality of their feelings, so that they do not fear losing their mind as a result of the experience.

7 Allow for individual differences, once more providing reassurance about the range of responses and ways of coping.
8 Give access to longer term, non-intensive support.
9 Explore coping styles, in particular the use of potentially maladaptive methods such as alcohol misuse.
10 Identify unresolved grief and take steps to provide further help when necessary.

In the context of AIDS, reading material prepared by those with practical experience in dealing with the consequences of the infection can help to anticipate problems and to reduce the sense of isolation. Martelli (1987), Sims and Moss (1991) and Kirkpatrick (1993) are examples of books with useful practical information which can help prevent problems.

Psychotropic medication is usually not indicated in the majority of cases of uncomplicated grief. However, short-term use of hypnotics to allow the grieving person to have the chance to rest at night, and so have the opportunity to continue adapting to the loss, may be of value if there is severe and persistent insomnia.

Management of Pathological Grief

As quoted above, it has been estimated that as many as 20% of bereaved individuals experience pathological grief (Jacobs 1993), and some pointers towards identifying such individuals have been described (Lazare 1979). The variety of pathological grief reactions and the range of personal and cultural differences that exist suggest that there is no simple, universal approach to dealing successfully with pathological grief, and that it will be important to tailor the intervention to the specific problems and needs of each particular bereaved person. Psychological interventions will sometimes need to be complemented by the use of psychopharmacological approaches, in particular when grief is associated with psychiatric disorders.

Psychological Interventions

A variety of psychological treatments, including both individual and family modalities, have been used in pathological grief (see Jacobs (1993) for review of studies). The majority of specific interventions that have been the subject of outcome research are of relatively brief duration, usually around three or four months. This does not mean that in all cases, psychological intervention is effective in such a rapid way. In practice, grief therapy can be a lengthy procedure, requiring a range of therapeutic skills and approaches.

Individual crisis intervention approaches. These focus on the expression of grief and have been shown to be effective for people at risk of complicated grief (Raphael 1977), while family-based crisis intervention has not been shown to be effective (Williams and Polak 1979).

Behavioural therapies. As in the case of guided mourning (Mawson, Marks and Ramm 1981), these are effective in dealing with the features of unresolved grief, in particular its avoidant behavioural aspects.

Brief psychodynamic individual psychotherapy. This has been shown (Marmar, Horowitz and Weiss 1988) to be as effective as peer-support groups, but the study did not include a no or minimal treatment group.

There are shared elements in the various forms of psychological intervention, even when the focus of therapy is different. Jacobs (1993) highlights the psychoeducational elements in grief therapy which lead to exposure to the feelings, behaviours and cognitions that tend to prolong mourning. Achieving the tasks of mourning described by Worden (1992) in relation to normal grief also applies to its pathological forms, although the process is likely to be much more complex.

When pathological grief is associated with psychiatric syndromes, such as PTSD, depression or anxiety disorders, specific psychological interventions for these disorders will be required (Gelder, Gath and Mayou 1989), although the feelings and thoughts being dealt with will be related to the loss.

Psychopharmacological Interventions

There has been no systematic research on the use of psychopharmacological treatments for pathological grief, and what knowledge there is rests basically on clinical experience.

Hypnotic medication. This, usually in the form of benzodiazepines, is recommended in cases of persistent insomnia of the kind that contributes to making the bereaved person exhausted and less able to focus on the tasks of mourning. It is important to stress to the bereaved that medication is not being used to suppress feelings or avoid exposure to painful memories, but rather to enable the person to deal more effectively with such distressing experiences. Hypnotics are usually required for only short periods of time, commonly in the early stages of mourning.

Antidepressant medication. This may be necessary in some cases of pathological grief, in particular those with marked depressive symptoms and signs and with a tendency to chronicity (Gelder, Gath and Mayou 1989). Antidepressant medication is unlikely to be effective in minimizing sadness when it is not part of a psychiatric disorder, and so it is important to carry out an adequate mental state examination before deciding on the use of antidepressants for bereaved people.

Sedatives. These are seldom required in the management of pathological grief, although they may be of value when used for a short time in cases of acute, severe grief, together with psychological treatments, such as crisis intervention.

Other Psychiatric Interventions

Pathological grief associated with psychiatric disorders may sometimes require the use of approaches familiar to psychiatrists, such as hospitalization or the use of other physical methods of treatment, such as ECT for severe depression. Clearly, what is being treated in such cases is not so much the pathological grief, but its psychiatric manifestations.

Peer or Mutual Support Interventions

In many developed countries there has been a rediscovery in recent years of the value of informal social supports to deal with many life problems. Such a development may well be a response to the demographic and social changes resulting from urban lifestyles and the disappearance of extended families. There is evidence that support groups can be very helpful to bereaved individuals, possibly reaching people who might not be in contact with professional services (see Jacobs (1993) for review).

Community-based mutual support groups have been an important feature of the HIV epidemic in developing countries, and it is fair to say that the range of services provided by such support groups could not have been matched by professional statutory agencies (Arno 1986; Williams 1988). Bereavement counselling services for people affected by HIV infection have been an integral part of such services, often working in collaboration with professional and statutory services (Sims and Moss 1991, Kirkpatrick 1993). See Chapters 2, 5 and 6 for more details.

CONCLUSION

The special features of the HIV epidemic – stigma and guilt associated with the disease, protracted physical decline, loss of young lives, exposure to multiple bereavement, to name a few – can lead to the development of complicated pathological grief disorders in those involved in the lives of people with HIV infection. Against these features and often in response to an unsympathetic and rejecting environment, the last decade has seen the development of new models of care to help people with HIV infection and their relatives and partners. Collaboration between statutory and voluntary agencies has been a crucial element of these new approaches. It is very likely that such joint efforts have contributed significantly to facilitate the process of grieving for the extensive loss of lives caused by HIV infection. However, the repeated exposure to deaths of patients, partners or simply acquaintances continues to represent a major challenge for all those touched by HIV infection.

REFERENCES

American Psychiatric Association (1987) *Diagnostic and Statistical Manual of Mental Disorders: 3rd edn. Revised* (DSM–III–R). Washington DC: APA

Arno PS (1986) The non-profit sector's response to the AIDS epidemic: Community-based services in San Francisco *Am J Publ Health* **76**: 1325–30

Bowlby J (1977a) The making and breaking of affectional bonds – I *Br J Psychiatry* **130**: 201–10

Bowlby J (1977b) The making and breaking of affectional bonds – II *Br J Psychiatry* **130**: 421–31

Bowlby J (1980) *Attachment and Loss: Loss, Sadness and Depression* New York: Basic Books

Clayton PJ (1990) Bereavement and depression *J Clin Psychiatry* **51**: 34–8

Deutsch H (1937) Absence of grief *Psychoanal Q* **6**: 12–22

Engel GL (1961) Is grief a disease? A challenge for medical research *Psychosom Med* **23**: 18–22

Freud S (1917) Mourning and melancholia. In *Standard Edition of the Complete Psychological Works of Sigmund Freud* London: Hogarth Press vol XIV

Gelder M, Gath D & Mayou R (1989) *Oxford Textbook of Psychiatry 2nd edn* Oxford: Oxford Medical Publications

Jacobs S (1993) *Pathologic Grief: Maladaptation to Loss* Washington DC: American Psychiatric Press

Jacobs SC, Hansen FF, Berkman L et al (1989) Depressions of bereavement *Compr Psychiatry* **30**: 218–24

Jacobs SC, Hansen FF, Kasl SV et al (1990) Anxiety disorders during acute bereavement: risk and risk factors *J Clin Psychiatry* **51**: 269–74

Kirkpatrick W (1993) *AIDS: Sharing the Pain* London: Darton Longman and Todd

Kubler-Ross E (1969) *On Death and Dying* New York: Macmillan

Lazare A (1979) Unresolved grief. In A Lazare (ed) *Outpatient Psychiatry: Diagnosis and Treatment* Baltimore: Williams and Wilkins pp 498–512

Lindemann E (1944) Symptomatology and management of acute grief *Am J Psychiatry* **101**: 141–8

Marmar C, Horowitz M & Weiss D (1988) A controlled trial of brief psychotherapy and mutual help group treatment of conjugal bereavement *Am J Psychiatry* **145**: 203–9

Martelli LJ (1987) *When someone you know has AIDS* New York: Crown Publishers

Mawson D, Marks I & Ramm L (1981) Guided mourning for morbid grief: a controlled study *Br J Psychiatry* **138**: 185–93

Parkes CM (1970) The first year of bereavement: a longitudinal study of the reaction of London widows to the death of husbands *Psychiatry* **33**: 444–67

Parkes CM (1972) *Bereavement Studies of Grief in Adult Life* New York: International Universities Press

Raphael B (1977) Preventive intervention with the recently bereaved *Arch Gen Psychiatry* **34**: 1450–4

Raphael B (1983) *The Anatomy of Bereavement* New York: Basic Books

Reite M & Field T (eds) *The Psychobiology of Attachment and Separation* New York: Academic Press

Sims R & Moss V (1991) *Terminal Care for People with AIDS* London: Edward Arnold

Williams MJ (1988) Gay men as 'buddies' to persons living with AIDS and ARC *Smith Coll Stud Soc Work* **59**: 38–52

Williams W & Polak P (1979) Follow-up research in primary prevention *J Clin Psychol* **135**: 35–45

Worden JW (1992) *Grief Counselling and Grief Therapy: a Handbook for the Mental Health Practitioner* London: Routledge

CHAPTER 5

Grief and the Community

Janet Seeley

MRC, Entebbe, Uganda

and

Ellen B. Kajura

MRC, Entebbe, Uganda

Sister Ursula Sharpe, a medical missionary working in South West Uganda, has described the last six years in Uganda as 'one long grieving period' as a result of AIDS-related mortality (Sharpe 1993). A reporter in *The Independent* (Calder 1993) portrayed this sense of tragedy in the following way:

> . . . Between the hymns the preacher struck up a sombre tone: 'those of you who have not yet mourned, prepare to mourn'. This was not fiery evangelism, just a reflection of awful reality. Even in the middle of a happy Sunday, under a bountiful sun, one disease casts a mortal shadow on this country. Almost every family has been touched by AIDS. Uganda sometimes feels like a condemned nation . . .

This chapter will draw on experience gained through work with the MRC/ODA/UVRI Research Programme on AIDS in Uganda, a long-term multidisciplinary, population-based research programme,[1] together with information gained from other commentators, to explore some aspects of grief in the community in Africa.

Uganda, as an African country, provides many examples. Current estimates of HIV infection rates in Uganda range from 20 to 30% among young, urban adults while rural rates tend to vary from 3 to 12% (Nkowane 1991; Serwadda, Wawer and Musgrave 1992). In the 15 villages in Masaka District, South West Uganda, which make up the study area of the MRC/ODA/UVRI Programme in Uganda (total population 10 000 people), young adults infected with HIV-1 have a risk of dying which is

Grief and AIDS. Edited by L. Sherr.
©1995 John Wiley & Sons Ltd.

60 times the risk of the non-infected. Half of all adult deaths and more than 80% of deaths in young adults are associated with HIV-1 (Mulder et al 1994). One elderly resident in the area commented that 'our children are sick mainly with AIDS and many have died. Every week we expect to bury one'.

UNAFFECTED, AFFLICTED AND AFFECTED

Barnett and Blaikie (1992: 86) categorize three types of household: 'unaffected' households in which no member is ill or has died from AIDS and which has not been affected by the illness or death of a member of any related household; 'afflicted' households where a member of the household is either ill or has died from the disease; 'affected' households that have been affected by the disease either through the death of a family (not necessarily a household) member who was contributing cash, labour or other support, or because the death of a family member has meant that orphans have joined the household. In the MRC study area in Masaka District, and in neighbouring Rakai District (part of which was the focus of Barnett and Blaikie's research), there are very few unaffected households and many households at different times are both afflicted and affected.[2]

THE SOCIAL BURDEN

The AIDS epidemic places a burden upon the formal and informal social security systems in Uganda, systems which were only just beginning to recover from two decades of war, civil unrest, economic decline and social disintegration. Like the recent wars and civil unrest in Uganda, HIV infection is claiming the lives of many able-bodied young people, but as Barnett and Blaikie (1992: 55) observe: 'AIDS differs in some crucial respects from other types of disaster . . . the AIDS pandemic does not take the form of a discrete event with recognizable stages and responses'. After 'natural' disasters it may be possible for communities to grieve together, and in the aftermath of war communal grieving may be focused on an 'armistice day' or, as in Uganda, a 'heroes day' when those who lost their lives in battle may be remembered and their deaths honoured. For the many people who have died and continue to die from AIDS-related infections there are few acts of 'communal grieving'; attempts have been made to make time to remember those who have died: the 'Names Project' with the memorial quilt begun in the United States of America and acts of observance around World Aids Day at the beginning of December are cases in point.

For many families the pain of loss due to death and the grieving process is compounded by the stigma that continues to be associated with HIV/AIDS. This stigma is shared by the family with their member or members who have died.

COMMUNITY ATTITUDES IN AFRICA TO HIV/AIDS-RELATED MORBIDITY AND MORTALITY

In view of the scale of the epidemic in Africa, where WHO predicts that by the year 2000 a cumulative total of 15 to 20 million people will have been infected (WHO 1990), it may be hoped that people are coming to terms with the effects of the sickness and death. Some commentators have suggested that there has been an under-reaction to AIDS in Africa. Ankrah (1991: 970), for example, comments: 'The fact that there is no cure for AIDS has unwittingly programmed the minds of people to become uncommonly tolerant of death. Even the most robust and promising of young Africans may accept as inevitable that their deaths are imminent'. Caldwell, Orubuloye and Caldwell (1992: 1178) agree with this view, which they attribute to beliefs in predestination and ' a strong belief in survival after death in one form or another'. Indeed, Sister Ursula (Sharpe 1993) said: 'In Uganda the word to die means to change: life does not end but changes'. In an ethnography of the Baganda, described in Roscoe (1965: 98) it was said: 'Death from natural causes rarely presented itself to the native mind as a feasible explanation for the end of life; illness was much more likely to be the result of malice finding vent in magical art'. But do such beliefs make death from AIDS understandable or even bearable?

Young people in our study were fond of quoting proverbs in discussions about AIDS. The common saying 'Will they saw timber out of me?' was interpreted to mean that the speaker believed that he or she was already infected, or at risk of being infected, with HIV; life would therefore be short and nothing would be gained from trying to alter behaviour to live longer. One 21-year-old woman, when discussing difficulties in changing behaviour, said:

> When one loses relatives many times then one loses hope. One thinks one could have an accident and die in a few days anyway, so why worry. So she decides to be social before she dies. One says 'I have never had a child yet this disease is taking many friends. How can I die without ever having produced?' Some fear not having a grandchild to keep their memory, so she gives herself up for birth.

When conversation turned to the number of people infected in Uganda people would say things like 'Oh, we are all going to die'. If told that many more people in the study area were free of infection than were infected (and that something needed to be done to protect those people) people would be full of disbelief, convinced that there must be some mistake. Counsellors in the study area have had clients for HIV testing coming back again and again, convinced that their negative test result was false. They were sure that they must be infected. However, when discussion turned to personal risk of infection people tended not to see themselves as at risk. They would comment: 'I'm safe and so are my people, but the others . . .' (Huygens et al 1994).

MOURNING RITES AND BURIAL

Roscoe (1965: 98–127) recounts the many rituals and obligations surrounding death and burial in Uganda. He describes lengthy periods of mourning, of two to six months for a chief and a month for an ordinary male household head, during which time relatives could not work. Even for a small child a burial was followed by two days of mourning for the relatives after which the mother would mourn alone for an assigned period. Death was costly, therefore, not only in terms of the person lost but also for the work time taken in observing all the rites. However, today the amount of time spent mourning has decreased considerably, largely because of a recognition that with the number of deaths occurring no work would ever be done if everyone mourned for the traditional time period. AIDS is held to be responsible for the increase in deaths. One 65-year-old woman in our study area commented that 'people are no longer scared of death. When they hear one has died, they keep on with their business. They mind about their field work first'. Ankrah (1993: 16) makes a similar observation:

> The practice now is to keep the bereaved company on the night of death or the arrival of the body, assist with preparing the grave, feed the mourners and attend the funeral.

But even though the 'mourning time' may be shorter, villagers in the study area, as in other parts of Uganda, are still very concerned to fulfil their customary obligations to the dead person, in the same way that they expect to be treated when they die. Thus, work continues to be disrupted by the periods of one or two days when household members cannot dig, or do other tasks, when a relative or neighbour has just died (Seeley 1993: 62–3). Such times of mourning are important because as Barnett and Blaikie (1992: 13) comment: 'In all societies and for most ordinary people, children and funerals are the only exception they may have of surviving in people's memories beyond the grave'.

Traditionally 'neighbours, kinsmen and significant other mourners were expected to contribute to funeral costs, including food' (Ankrah 1993: 15). There was and still is the hope of reciprocity. Ainsworth and Rwegarulira (1991) observe that in rural Tanzania even households not experiencing an adult death feel the impact of the epidemic indirectly because they will be asked to contribute to the funerals of their neighbours and relatives, assist with health care costs, the care of the sick and children and perhaps help with fieldwork. Thus, not surprisingly, the financial and other demands on family and neighbours have become a significant burden because of the multiple deaths from AIDS.

In many places in Africa (and elsewhere) 'funeral associations' have existed in the past, made up of clan members who provide financial and emotional support to each other at times of death. In Rakai and Masaka Districts in Uganda these groups are termed Munno Mu Kabi (literally 'friend in need') and there have been efforts in some places to build on these structures to provide local support groups for communities hard hit by AIDS-related deaths.[3] However, it is evident that multiple loss is putting an intolerable strain on many families and communities. The hope that support may be received from family and friends is now not always realized. One example comes from a family that had suffered its third loss in two months:

> Lydia complained that when she had sent for her sons in Kampala to come and help her with Sara's (co-wife who was ill in Kampala) dying daughter they had refused to come. She told the interviewer that she wondered what was wrong with relatives nowadays that they did not assist their family in times of need. Neighbours had helped her to lay out the body and then prepare for the funeral.

It could well be that after a series of deaths the other relatives, as well as Lydia herself, were feeling the strain of coping with the burden of care.

It must be remembered that the financial and emotional burden of death and burial often follows weeks and months of caring for the sick person. Although burials and funeral rites take up villagers' time and usually involve some financial contribution to the ceremony, tending the sick also 'costs' time and money. Unlike the time taken on the 'rites of passage' ceremonies, the time spent taking care of ill relatives is usually unpredictable and can mean weeks rather than days away from duties and other responsibilities.

GRIEF COMPOUNDED BY ECONOMIC HARDSHIP

Caring for a child, partner, relative or friend who is going to die imposes a great emotional and often financial burden on a household. This burden may be further compounded by the loss of an important income earner, or potential income earner, for the home. In Zimbabwe, as in other parts of Africa, many households in the rural areas have become dependent upon remittances sent from members (often husbands, sons and daughters) working in urban areas or on commercial farms. The impact of sickness and death from HIV-related infections and substantial price rises as a result of structural adjustment pose substantial threats to this support structure.[4]

A counsellor gave the following account of the reaction to the death of a son in a poor farming family:

> In this home a son died of AIDS at a time when his father was expecting a lot out of him. The old man said sadly that he had lost the heir to the home because he did not have another child like that son. The family was upset by the fact that this boy had left no child. One of the boy's sisters said 'he left no picture of him in the world, so we have completely lost him'.

This family not only felt the loss of the boy but also the loss of his potential children, his heirs.

Ngugi (1992: 56) tells a similar story of grief mixed with disappointment. A 26-year-old man in Bukoba, Tanzania had to return from further study overseas because he had HIV-related infections:

> One of Gregory's major worries was how to deal with his parents, who had already started traditional mourning . . . Living in a patriarchal society, they were deeply ashamed and disappointed that their only son had AIDS and that their investment for their old age had been demolished. That is why they mourned while Gregory was still alive.

Children, as well as parents and siblings, pay a high price when fathers, mothers, uncles and aunts die prematurely. School fees may no longer be available and household tasks may fall heavily upon their shoulders. They as orphans may find themselves a burden for relatives struggling to care for their own families. They may also forfeit their anticipated inheritance. Two Ugandan households illustrate this:

> The head of a poor household, Varista, spent nearly 10 000/-[5] over a period of two months attending first the burial and then the last funeral rites of her father. For her father's funeral, as was her customary obligation, she had to make a contribution to the ceremony. She complained bitterly that her father, who had been ill for five years, had used up all of his resources seeking treatment and there was nothing left for her and her siblings to inherit.

> Harriet, another poor householder, spent two months tending her dying husband. She said that her main reason for going back to take care of him,

a man she had left because he was cruel to her, was to ensure that her children retained their rights to their father's property. She, too, was disappointed. He had used up nearly all his money on seeking treatment for his illnesses which, according to Harriet, were due to AIDS.

'Africa's high and increasing number of children left without the care of one or both parents, called by some "AIDS orphans", is one of the most striking outcomes of the AIDS epidemic' (Ankrah 1993: 16). For elderly relatives the grief associated with the loss of their child(ren) and the shock of perhaps losing their anticipated source of security in their declining years, is compounded by the burden of caring for their children's children. AIDS has been called 'the grandmother's burden' (Beer, Rose and Tout 1988) and there has been considerable publicity given to the plight of elderly women left with numerous children to care for (Perlez 1990). There are many stories of mothers who pay a high emotional price through nursing their adult children until death and then find themselves hard-pressed to pick up the pieces of their household livelihood and maintain a home for their orphaned grandchildren.

GRIEF AND LONELINESS

In addition to the loss of financial support, there is often a considerable emotional impact resulting from a death. One household head in Uganda, a 30-year-old woman, often complained to a counsellor that she was lonely. Her sister, who had been the previous household head, had died in 1990 and she was left with her sister's two children and a child of her brother to care for. Moreover, the children caused problems for their aunt because she found them difficult to control, but when they were at school she complained that she was lonely. She often told the interviewer about the loss of 'her relatives who have died at an early age of AIDS and did not live to see any reward for their hard work'. In December 1991 the woman's cousin came to stay to help her to organize a New Year's party. A visitor at that time commented: 'Regina was so excited and in the happiest mood that I have ever seen [her in] because she had a visitor of her own age'.

Loneliness is commonly associated with grief, the loneliness arising both from the loss of a 'special' person to interact with and from a lack of company in general (Littlewood 1992: 45). Where multiple losses from AIDS occur individuals may find their 'healing web of friends and relatives' (Van den Boom and Gremmen 1992) severely depleted and they may find that grief is exacerbated by the lack of someone to share with, as in the case above.

The economic and emotional loss can be aggravated by society's attitude towards those who die from HIV/AIDS-related disease.

AIDS-RELATED STIGMA

On a global scale there is increasing discrimination against people with HIV infection. Family members are also affected by social stigma and may experience rejection from friends, loss of jobs and harassment. (Bor, Miller and Goldman 1993: 191).

Social stigma remains a serious burden for HIV-positive persons and their families studied in Uganda. Just before a 30-year-old woman died of AIDS-related sicknesses in one of the villages she remarked to a visitor:

I feel that even good people when they are being nice to me, all the time . . . underneath they look at me as a wrong doer. That is how they see it and they are not able to accept me as anything else.

In a study on the care given to 30 sick counselling clients it was found that care was limited, or denied, by clients' families because of stigma. In three cases the patient was subjected to ridicule by relatives who blamed her (in all three cases the patient was female) for her condition (Seeley et al 1993). The blaming of people with HIV/AIDS-related sicknesses for their condition has been widely reported. Kegeles et al (1989), for example, observe that 'many Americans continue to stigmatize people with AIDS, perceiving them to be deserving of the disease as punishment for offensive or immoral behavior'.

The stigma of AIDS may lead people to try to disassociate themselves from the disease when a family member or neighbour has died. It is common practice in parts of Uganda for people at a burial to be given a short account of the deceased's life and the cause of death. It continues to be unusual for 'AIDS-related infections' to be cited as a cause of death; people commonly say 'headache', 'fever', even 'typhoid' in much the same way that obituaries in Europe and North America talk of 'death after a long illness'. Muyindwa et al (1993) tell the following story of denial after a man's wife had died of AIDS-related illnesses:

One Silasi, a resident of one of the study villages, lost his wife and I paid a visit to him one evening. After welcoming me I gave him my condolences for the loss of his wife. 'Ah no, she was just a porter. She was not my wife . . . ' Silasi replied. This is the Silasi who invited people to attend the wedding when marrying the deceased . . . now Silasi disowned her as his wife.

For many people, grieving for their lost family member is complicated by the fear of the disease and the very real concerns of partners that they may also be infected. An 18-year-old woman commented: 'In Baganda there is a saying "Tell me who you walk with and I will tell you your behaviour''. If people are friends and one of them gets AIDS, others fear to associate with the one infected, for they may be thought to have AIDS too' (Muyindwa et al 1993).

MULTIPLE LOSSES, THE IMPACT ON THE FAMILY AND COMMUNITY

Sickness and death are testing the ability of many communities in Africa and elsewhere, to cope. A number of commentators have remarked that in Uganda multiple losses from AIDS-related deaths are added to the often bitter recent history:

> Over the past decade, Uganda has been saddled with the bloody military rule of dictator Idi Amin followed by civil strife and guerilla war that have destroyed much of the country's social, economic and political fabric. The AIDS epidemic is the latest in the series of scourges that have hit the nation. (Kisekka 1990: 35)

While courageous efforts are being made by some to cope with the economic and emotional cost inflicted by the epidemic many people, in particular women, continue to fear the stigma associated with HIV infection and cover their grief in the activity of rebuilding their homes and livelihoods. Some, who know (or fear) themselves to be infected, wonder how they will cope with the debilitating illnesses from which they see husbands, brothers, sisters and other relatives suffering.

The first concern of most people is, however, the future well-being of their children. For example, an HIV-positive counselling client, a widow, was living with her own children and was doing relatively well out of the produce of her land. She was still healthy and was reluctant to tell her relatives about her HIV status for fear of stigma. However, she told the counsellor that other relatives were pressing her to take the children of a deceased brother into her home. She confided that she was reluctant to do so because she wanted to save her resources for her own children in preparation for her own decline and death. Her relatives could not understand why she was refusing to take the children, whom she could clearly, in their eyes, afford to keep.

A PLACE FOR COUNSELLING AND SUPPORT SERVICES

Seeley et al (1991) have described how a counselling component was established to provide a support structure for villagers wishing to know their HIV status. This service, provided by village-based counsellors drawn from the local population, has broadened into a general community support service that aims to strengthen local people's ability to help themselves and others (Seeley et al 1994). Because the counsellors are local people whose own lives are affected by AIDS-related sickness and death, they have experience to share with people coping with HIV in their own families. Providing support at times of grief is often difficult. Counsellors may have to cope with a family resentful that medicine (both 'traditional' and 'Western') failed to save the life of their lost family member or with people fearful of their own HIV status who may react to the death of a wife or husband by denying that AIDS was involved. If a counsellor has had time to build up a relationship with a client's family and perhaps neighbourhood through periods of illness, there is a chance that fears and prejudices will have been aired and the consequences of impending death explored.

The emphasis has been upon *community*-based counselling in recognition of the fact that HIV/AIDS is one factor among many that influence the lives of people in rural areas in Uganda, as in most places. Economic, social, perhaps political factors may impinge upon the way people react to HIV infection and death. By encouraging family and community members to discuss AIDS, by providing information and by giving practical examples of care, counsellors have an opportunity to reduce the stigma attached to AIDS and in a way make the lives of affected families easier.

At times of death the counsellors have sometimes found that they are warmly welcomed by the grieving family because they are 'people who understand' and do not fear association with families touched by HIV. When a counsellor visited a home where a young man had just died the mother expressed this sentiment in the following way:

> I know my child would have died long ago if it was not for the doctors. But I especially want to thank you [the local counsellor] for the love and concern you expressed when my son was ill. You always visited us and made us comfortable even with the many problems of nursing my son.

CONCLUSION

Stigma and denial continue to haunt communities in Uganda and other parts of Africa where every household is affected by HIV infection and death and there are enormous barriers for coping with the grief inflicted by the many deaths. However, something positive may come out of this atmosphere of fear. A lead is shown by some courageous individuals and families who have suffered and wish to help others, for example, Noreen Kaleeba, one of the founders of the AIDS Support Organization (TASO).

. . . .

Rita was a young woman who had recently died in her home. During the previous four years she had nursed her older sister until death (from AIDS-related infections) and as a community counsellor had helped numerous clients in practical ways as well as providing a sympathetic ear for their troubles. From her example some other young people learned how to cope with the loss of their friends and the threat that HIV infection posed to their lives. There are many Ritas and would-be Ritas in Urganda. Rita's example of sharing and caring and fighting the stigma of HIV infection, provides a way forward for the many grieving people in communities all over the world who are counting the ever-increasing economic and emotional cost of AIDS.

. . . .

ACKNOWLEDGEMENTS

The authors are grateful to the MRC/ODA/UVRI Programme staff for their contributions to this work. Helpful comments and suggestions were made by seminar participants when earlier versions of this chapter were presented at the Department of Anthropology, University College London and Department of Social Anthropology, University of Cambridge; that assistance is gratefully acknowledged.

The Director, Uganda Virus Research Institute, and Director of Medical Services, Ministry of Health, are thanked for their support and for permission to publish this work.

NOTES

1 The Programme was established in 1988 at the invitation of the Ugandan Government with the primary aim of studying the population dynamics of HIV-1 transmission and associated risk factors in a rural population. The Programme, funded by MRC/ODA (UK Government) up until mid–1998, works in collaboration with the Uganda Virus Research Institute of the Ugandan Ministry of Health.
2 In 1991/1992 the MRC Programme conducted a small study of HIV infection in Lukaya, a town on the trans-African highway close to the MRC study area. It was found that the adult HIV prevalence is 40% and that 65% of households (98/154) had at least one infected adult at the time of the study.
3 The work of the Irish charity Concern in Rakai District, Uganda is one example, where the expatriate workers are helping local communities to strengthen Munno Mu Kabi groups so that they not only have the capacity to help each other at funerals but also through times of sickness and other problems. In the MRC study area similar initiatives are under way (Kajura et al 1993).

4 Ken Wilson (Ford Foundation, Harare) October 1993, personal communication.
5 At that time there were about 1000/- to the $1. Varista's usual monthly income was in the region of 1000/- or 2000/- depending upon whether she has surplus crops to sell, or perhaps a chicken. When she needed extra cash, for travel or for paying for health care, she would raise money by brewing some beer, digging someone else's land or selling some chickens or perhaps get some money from a friend.

REFERENCES

Ainsworth M & Rwegarulira AA (1991) Coping with the AIDS epidemic in Tanzania: survivor assistance *Background paper prepared for the Tanzania AIDS Assessment and Planning Study, World Bank*, Washington DC

Ankrah EM (1991) AIDS and the social side of health *Soc Sci Med* **32**: 967–80

Ankrah EM (1993) The impact of HIV/AIDS on the family and other significant relationships: the African clan revisited. *AIDS Care* **5**(1): 5–22

Barnett T & Blaikie P (1992) *AIDS in Africa: Its Present and Future Impact* London: Belhaven Press

Beer C, Rose A & Tout K (1988) AIDS – the grandmother's burden. In AF Fleming et al (eds) *The Global Impact of AIDS* New York: Alan R Liss pp 171–4

Bor R, Miller R & Goldman E (1993) HIV/AIDS and the family: a review of research in the first decade *J Fam Ther* **15**: 187–204

Calder S (1993) Down here in heaven *The Independent* 16 October: 37

Caldwell JC, Orubuloye IO & Caldwell P (1992) Underreaction to AIDS in Sub-Saharan Africa *Soc Sci Med* **34**: 1169–82

Huygens P, Kajura E, Seeley J & Mulder D (1994) Rethinking methods for studying sexual behaviours: questioning questioning (forthcoming)

Kajura E, Nabaitu C, Bachengana et al (1993) Building community capacity to cope with adversity: the role of traditional support networks *VIII Int Con AIDS in Africa* (Marrakesh)

Kegeles SM, Coates TJ, Christopher TA & Lazarus JL (1989) Perception of AIDS: the continuing saga of AIDS-related stigma *AIDS* **3**: (suppl 1): S253–8

Kisekka MN (1990) AIDS in Uganda as a gender issue. In ED Rothblum & E Cole (eds) *Women's Mental Health in Africa* New York: Haworth Press pp 35–53

Littlewood J (1992) *Aspects of Grief. Bereavement in Adult Life* London: Routledge

Mulder DW, Nunn AJ, Kamali A et al (1993) HIV-1 associated mortality in a rural population in Uganda: results after two years follow up (forthcoming)

Muyindwa H, Sembajja F, Seeley J et al (1993) Social aspects of AIDS related stigma in rural areas *Working Paper* Entebbe: MRC/ODA Research Programme on AIDS in Uganda

Ngugi E (1992) Caring: the cost to a community. In *The Hidden Cost of AIDS: Challenge of HIV to Development* London: Panos Publications p 56

Nkowane BM (1991) Prevalence and incidence of HIV infection in Africa: a review of data published in 1990 *AIDS* **5** (suppl 1): S7–15

Perlez J (1990) In Uganda district, AIDS orphans struggle to survive *New York Times* 10 June

Roscoe J (1965) *The Baganda. An Account of their Native Customs and Beliefs* 2nd edn London: Frank Cass

Seeley J (1993) *Searching for Indicators of Vulnerability. A Study of Household Coping Strategies in Rural South West Uganda* Entebbe: MRC/ODA Research Programme on AIDS in Uganda

Seeley J, Kajura E, Bachengana C et al (1993) The extended family and support for people with AIDS in a rural population in SW Uganda. A safety net with holes? *Aids Care* **5**(1): 121–6

Seeley JA, Wagner U, Mulemwa J et al (1991) The development of a community based HIV/AIDS counselling service in a rural area in Uganda *AIDS Care* **3**(2) 211–21

Seeley J, Balmer DH, Kengeya-Kayondo JF & Mulder DW (1994) Can the jigsaw puzzle fit together? Participatory research, community development, counselling and sustainability in a community based HIV/AIDS research programme in rural Uganda (forthcoming)

Serwadda D, Wawer MJ & Musgrave SD (1992) HIV risk factors in three geographic strata of rural Rakai District, Uganda *AIDS* **6**: 983–9

Sharpe U (1993) The 1993 Pope Paul VI Memorial Lecture, Leeds *AIDS Newsletter* **8**(12): 11 (item 742)

Van den Boom F & Gremmen AW (1992) AIDS and grief *VIII Int Con AIDS* (Amsterdam) Poster PoB 3814

World Health Organization (WHO) (1990) *Current and Future Dimensions of the HIV/AIDS Pandemic* Geneva: WHO/GPA

CHAPTER 6

AIDS Health Care: Staff Stress, Loss and Bereavement

Lydia Bennett

The University of Sydney, Australia

The experiences of grief and bereavement are substantially documented in people living with HIV/AIDS, their relatives, lovers and friends. However, the influence of grief and bereavement on health care professionals has received relatively scant attention. A unique aspect of AIDS-related care is that many health care providers *are* relatives, lovers and friends. The experience of losing people with AIDS from close relationships while acting as care providers for them has been reported by health care providers as an emotionally taxing combination (Bennett 1992a,b).

There are possible yet unclear links and interactions between the experiences of stress, burnout, loss and grief in the area of AIDS health care. These links will be explored to ascertain who may be vulnerable, the nature of the relationship, how to predict and prevent staff stress and grief and how to intervene in situations where loss and burnout are being reported. A multitude of variables may contribute to the relationships between grief and stress. Health care professional role and status, personality, hours working in this area, relationships with clients, extent of identification with clients, recognition and reward and management styles may all influence the outcomes of working in this field.

Grief and AIDS. Edited by L. Sherr.
©1995 John Wiley & Sons Ltd.

GENERALIZATIONS FROM LITERATURE

Grief and Length of Time of Relationships with Patients

Why is it that some members of staff cope well with the losses associated with AIDS caregiving and others do not? Braybrook (1993: 15) states that 'the strength of the bond with the deceased person appears to be a strong predictor of the impact'. While this is recognized as an important variable in gay men, it needs to be emphasized in preparing *staff* for work in this field. The strength of the bond between staff and clients varies greatly, but in many units staff report it to be a strong and meaningful one (Martin 1990; Bennett 1992a,b; Gordon et al 1993).

The nature of AIDS-related admissions to hospital often involves repeated contact between patients and health care providers. This means that over an extended period of time the health care provider may spend more cumulative time with one patient than the average spent with a single patient in many other areas of health care. A staff member states that 'we get to know them all so well' (Bennett 1992b: 130). The length of time also helps to sanction the grieving associated with the loss. A nurse commented: 'If I have a long-term relationship with a patient it's more okay to talk about the loss. Length of time with a patient can give legitimacy to grieving' (Chapman Dick 1989: 62).

Emotional bonds, both positive and negative, investments of energy and interest, hopes and expectations are among the factors that give meaning and significance to a loss. The durability and intensity of these factors influence the perception of the loss (Baker and Kelly 1986). Because AIDS patients return repeatedly for care, staff become closely involved with intimate aspects of their patients' lives. The holistic model of care currently being practised in many units means that staff are involved in the management of psychosocial as well as physical aspects of the patients' care. Staff become very attached to patients during this process and this serves to intensify feelings of loss when their patients die.

In a study conducted by Martin (1990), the feelings of loss expressed by many of the nurses were more intense and enduring than had been anticipated. Martin explains this by the recurrent admissions of patients to the same units, resulting in nurses forming close relationships with patients. A further reason given by Martin (1990) is that, if a patient has been rejected by their family, the nurse seems to assume the role of a surrogate family member. Their sense of identification with the patient as well as grief over his or her death may have exceeded the expected feelings of frustration and loss associated with other types of terminally ill patients. Bennett (1992b: 130) quotes a respondent:

When they develop AIDS, all they experience is rejection until they encounter us, and we become the support for them, we become the family for them, which has never happened to me working in oncology.

In cases other than AIDS, the supports available to hospitalized patients usually include the family of origin, friends and neighbours. Christ and Wiener (1985) state that, for the majority of AIDS patients, the family of origin is less available and this causes a greater drain on others for support. Health care professionals become very important to the AIDS patient and greatly assist the patient in dealing with the stresses of the disease.

Hours Working in the Area and Experiences of Grief and Burnout

A number of studies have explored the influences on staff of the time that they have worked in the area. Burnout, for example, is rarely reported as occurring suddenly, but rather after a reasonable period of time on the job. In some studies, staff are more likely to report burnout after a longer period of time in their area of work (Bennett, Michie and Kippax 1991). Like burnout, grief is also predicted to have a stronger impact with greater length of time in the area. Bennett (1992b: 140) quotes a staff member:

> This disease is different to cancer, if your husband or your father has cancer the whole family can pull together and it's a one-off thing, but here it's flatmate upon flatmate . . . I guess for me that's the biggest difficulty with working here, watching the growing disease.

As the number of AIDS cases grows, so too will the strain on staff as they watch the increasing and devastating impact of this disease.

Horstman and McKusick (1986) found that for all the physicians in their study, the higher the percentage of time they spent in contact with AIDS patients, the more likely they were to experience psychological distress. AIDS practitioner stress and burnout appear to be more a function of concentrated exposure to, rather than longitudinal contact with, the disease. It appears that the intensity rather than chronicity of work contributes to AIDS health care worker morbidity.

Shulman and Mantell (1988: 982) state that 'health professionals have been overwhelmed by the daily confrontations with death . . .'. They explain how heavy physical care requirements, combined with the inevitable losing battle with death, create extraordinarily high levels of exhaustion and stress. House staff need to perform difficult and invasive procedures and social workers spend hours trying to help an AIDS patient to leave the acute facility, often with little or no success.

Maj (1991) cites the unpublished UK research, discussed by Miller (1988), which showed that the critical cutoff point for avoiding psychological distress was to spend less than 60% of the working week in the context of HIV-1 infection. While the ideal may be shorter hours of direct patient contact in AIDS health care, this is often not possible or practical to arrange. If staff are to spend long hours caring for people with AIDS, they need to be prepared for the emotional impact of frequent deaths.

Disenfranchised Grief

Doka (1989) introduced the concept of disenfranchised grief to assist the understanding of a loss that is not socially sanctioned. These are losses where a person does not have a clear, socially recognized right, role or capacity to grieve. The concept of disenfranchised grief recognizes that societies have sets of norms that specify who grieves for how long, where, when and how. In the disenfranchised griever, the person suffers a loss but has little or no opportunity to mourn publicly. In a society where most attention is placed on kin-based relationships and roles, it is not hard to foresee the difficulties of AIDS-related bereavement. The population of health care professionals working in the area of AIDS often experience grief that is disenfranchised. In the situation where staff are homosexual, they may face further isolation due to the negative sanction they face within the wider community.

Stigma and Discrimination

A study by Gordon and colleagues (1993) found that nurses working with AIDS received very little support from family and friends. It was suggested that this reflected society's stigmatization and avoidance of people associated with AIDS. Health care professionals may feel angry and despondent due to the discrimination they face. There is a loss of confidence and self-esteem when staff are judged according to their area of work or their HIV status. Their grief may be associated with the many losses they have had to face due to their choice of work area, and the unfairness of some losses is likely to intensify their feelings of grief.

RELATIONSHIPS BETWEEN ANXIETY, BURNOUT AND GRIEF

Price and Murphy (1984) compare burnout to loss and grief. They state that the understanding of grief has changed in the last two decades. It is no longer denoted as merely a state of sadness, but as a process that may embrace, over time, a range of internal states and overt behaviours, some of which are very different from weeping and sadness. Price and Murphy report that this has led to changed attitudes toward the grieving and bereaved persons, as well as increased capacities by many to recognize a variety of behaviours as coping modes in response to loss. Similarly, recognizing burnout as a process means that it can be intercepted and measured before it becomes severe, and treatment can be commenced early. It is necessary to recognize both the processes of burnout and grief in health care staff and to acknowledge and further explore the possible links between the two. A respondent in Bennett's study (1992b: 138) states:

> . . . in my first couple of months here, I thought burnout, what's burnout? . . . It was a good environment and nothing much happened until I started seeing people die en masse and people who I have nursed and who I've had quite a bit of interaction with, and then realising that I was starting to burn out . . .

In Bennett and Kelaher's study (1993a) anxiety was related to levels of grief. Respondents with a high level of grief were also more likely to score high on anxiety. The interactive relationship between grief and anxiety leads researchers to express concern about the influence that grief may have on health care professionals. If grief is not dealt with then staff may be more prone to burnout. Stroebe and Stroebe (1987) discuss the links between stress and grief to explain the physical and psychological consequences resulting from bereavement. They report that poor health, anxiety and inability to cope may result from multiple grief experiences.

Burnout as Adaptation to Loss

Price and Murphy (1984) state that burnout entails considerable loss for the worker and is, in part, a response to loss. The loss involved is described as a loss of an aspect of self which may include disillusionment, loss of motivation for creative involvement, and withdrawal from emotional aspects of relationships with clients and co-workers. Furthermore, relationships outside work may also be jeopardized. Price and Murphy (1984: 50) state that 'we feel confident in our judgement that high stress work with dying and bereaved persons puts one's intimate relationships at risk . . . burnout victims do not make good lovers'.

Price and Murphy (1984) cite Kavenaugh's (1973) seven stages of adaptation to stressful work, using professional care for the dying and bereaved as a framework for understanding this process. These seven stages are shock, disorganization, volatile emotions, guilt, loss and loneliness, relief and re-establishment.

The stages of shock and disorganization result from seeing patients die when carers are trained to cure and want to see people get better. The lack of focus on recovery may lead to a state of unreality and disorientation in the work setting. How health care professionals adapt to this may determine their emotional health and ability to accept death as a regular and anticipated outcome (Price and Murphy 1984).

Volatile emotions occur periodically for many staff during their work in terminal care. Support groups are necessary to provide empathy and acceptance of these emotions (Price and Murphy 1984). Years of conditioning may have taught that outward displays of emotion are childish and may result in staff suppressing their true feelings. Unless caregivers can express their emotions, there is no signal to alert others that support is required. Health care professionals are often good at giving, but are notoriously bad at receiving, support (Price and Murphy 1984).

Understanding and dealing with the stage of guilt is important to successful adaptation to loss. The death of a patient may result in a conscientious review of the standard of care that health care professionals have provided. Few can manage such a review without feeling some real or imagined failure to give the highest level of care. Gordon and colleagues (1993) reported that nurses who had been working with patients with haemophilia for 11 to 15 years were particularly vulnerable to feelings of guilt for having participated in the treatment that resulted in HIV infection. Learning to deal with feelings of guilt is important and has a considerable effect on the quality of future care provided.

Feeling guilty may act as a psychological antidote to feelings of helplessness, with thought processes such as 'if I am guilty, then I am responsible, and if I am responsible, then there is something I can do in the face of death' (Price and Murphy 1984: 54). Recognition of these processes for what they are enables staff to work with feelings of helplessness rather than carrying the load of guilt. Price and Murphy state that unexamined pseudoguilt and unforgiven real guilt are among the most destructive factors in the stress syndrome that may result in staff burnout.

Kavenaugh's stage of loneliness results when full awareness of the loss becomes a reality (1973). A persistent sharp sense of loneliness may be a signal for taking time off. A supportive environment can enable this pain to have a positive outcome as workers progress to a sound accommodation to their stressful work. Caregivers who cope with the above-mentioned stages may attain some sense of achievement in the realization that they survived this stress (Price and Murphy 1984). There is a sense of relief achieved through coping well. The adaptation that follows is a way of re-establishing balance in an altered environment. A positive outcome results in change that often involves enlarged personal capacities.

The stages of adaptation to a stressful work situation involving dying patients help us to understand the possible positive outcomes for workers who adapt to losses. They also warn us of variables that may lead to maladaptation, such as lack of expression of emotion and persistent, unresolved guilt.

ASPECTS OF DEATH CAUSING STAFF CONCERN

Staff interviewed about their experiences of caring in three Australian HIV/AIDS units reported perceptions and difficulties (Bennett 1992a). Death was the core category induced from qualitative analysis of the transcripts. Death and issues surrounding the deaths of patients were the greatest cause of concern for all health care workers. Seven aspects of death that were difficult or stressful were identified. These were: lack of a cure and all patients dying, the sheer number of deaths, feelings of powerlessness, relationships with patients and identification with patients, the nature of the deaths and the ethical dilemmas surrounding death. There were also positive aspects to caring for people dying from AIDS. Each of these aspects of death will be discussed in turn, in addition to references to other relevant research and literature.

Current Lack of a Cure

The first aspect of death causing staff distress and grief was the lack of a cure and the fact that all patients die. One female doctor said:

> The difficulty is that you know that eventually all these patients are going to die.

A female nurse commented:

> I guess the most significant difference is knowing that everyone you look after will die, whereas in other wards, even with someone who has maybe cancer or a renal disease, there's always maybe a little glimmer somewhere . . .

A male doctor states:

> The patients all die, so you have to change your perspective of the ward.

Nash (1985) cites Hingley's (1985) study in which nurses identified dealing with death and dying as a specific stressor, linked to the expectations that patients will be cured and restored to health by the medical profession. Ross and Seeger (1988) also found that respondents reported a sense of futility in treating these patients. There is clearly a need for staff to change their focus from cure to palliation.

The Number of Deaths and Responsibility for Death

Health care professionals are often unprepared for the impact of multiple experiences of grief and loss. These situations comprise more than the recognized losses associated with death and dying. Staff witness their clients losing weight and physical appearance, losing vitality and health, losing jobs, friends and living standards. All of these losses in clients have an impact on the carers who support them through this time.

Wolcott, Fawzy and Pasnau (1985) recognize that the high death rate in AIDS patients can result in repetitive grief reactions in staff members. Staff have just dealt with one death and another may occur. The large number of frequent deaths that are commonplace in some units do not allow the staff enough time or opportunity to grieve. Bolle (1988) and Piemme and Bolle (1990) warn that staff working in AIDS face 'bereavement overload'. This, they conclude, is caused by exposure to several terminally ill patients over a short period of time. A nurse reported (Bennett 1987: 1150–5):

> I lost 125 patients in about a year and a half . . . We are not prepared for this.

It may be that there is a cumulative effect of the high numbers of patients continually dying in the unit. A male doctor comments on how AIDS has had an impact on his life:

> Cumulatively, the deaths of the patients. I think I've killed about at least 40 people in hospital, about that many again have died outside of the hospital, and the one thing that I've noticed is that I'm getting angry at this disease – at the waste of people with the disease [pause] – sheer fury.

It seems that this doctor is taking responsibility for the deaths that have occurred as a result of AIDS/HIV. Price and Bergen (1977) revealed that health care professionals working in the stressful environment of a coronary care unit began to feel responsible for the lives of their patients. The professionals lost sight of the numerous extemporaneous factors that affect the patient in addition to the treatment. Wessells (1989) states that a professional would be better served to define success in terms of the quality of the process of their work as opposed to the outcome. The inability to cure patients may contribute to both the feelings of responsibility depicted by this doctor's phrase 'I've killed about at least 40 people', and feelings of anger and fury.

Identification with People Living with AIDS

Bennett (1992b) and Bennett and Kelaher (1993a) found that the intensity of experiences of grief and burnout were related to the levels of identification with clients. Staff who experienced higher levels of grief were those who reported higher identification with people with AIDS on self-report questionnaires (Bennett and Kelaher 1993a). This identification may place respondents at an emotional risk since they suffer more intense feelings of grief in response to patients' deaths.

Gay professionals may be more vulnerable to overidentification and may need to learn techniques to maintain a healthy distance from clients. However, this is not easy when many clients are already friends and when theirs is a close rapport because of similarities between the lives and experiences of professionals and clients.

Morin and Batchelor (1984) warn that the psychosocial issues facing gay professionals who are dealing with AIDS are immensely complex. They state that many will overidentify with people with AIDS and will push themselves too hard to provide care.

In the study by Horstman and McKusick (1986), physicians who identified themselves as gay were more likely than their heterosexual counterparts to have experienced increased anxiety, overwork, stress and fear of death since first working with AIDS. Interviews identified a number of factors to explain these results. Gay physicians' self-perception of being at risk for AIDS, and their identification with an ever increasing number of gay patients whose health status is deteriorating, both led to these differing responses.

Identification with patients was found to be an important factor contributing to grief and burnout in a study by Bennett (1992b). When respondents were asked about difficult or negative aspects of working with AIDS patients, many spoke about identification and referred to the additional problem of discerning the fine line between involvement and overinvolvement with patients. A respondent (1992b: 138) states that 'if you become overinvolved that's a rapid road to burnout'. Respondents who identify closely with their patients may need to be taught methods to maintain a healthy emotional distance in their work. It is difficult to know how to remain empathic and caring, while still protecting oneself from overinvolvement. Staff may benefit from time-out techniques, where they do something completely different from work to help separate their professional and private lives.

Powerlessness

A nurse in Bennett's study (1992a: 142) states that 'they're not going to get better and I feel powerless in any sort of intervention that I can do as a nurse'. Horstman and McKusick (1986) describe a syndrome occurring in physicians working with AIDS patients. Among the symptoms were depression, anxiety, hopelessness and general feelings of inadequacy.

They described the set of symptoms as the 'Helper Helplessness Syndrome'. To explore further what they had observed they measured anxiety, depression, overwork, stress and fear of death experienced by physicians engaged in AIDS-related professional activity. The majority reported more stress, and a significant minority reported more fear of death and anxiety since they had begun working with AIDS.

The Nature of Deaths and the Dilemmas of Palliation versus Aggressive Therapy

While staff find it difficult dealing with the deaths of young patients, a large proportion of staff said that the hardest aspect of their work was not the death itself but the nature of the deaths. A male nurse said:

> They die such hideous deaths.

Another male nurse (Bennett 1992a) commented:

> It's not so much death, because they don't talk a lot about that, it's that change in body image and hopelessness and the overwhelming disease . . .

Staff suffer stress in watching the changes in body image that lead to patients' death. In addition to this, staff also suffer stress, frustration and conflict surrounding the decisions made about death. A number of staff mention incidents and accounts of ethical dilemmas surrounding death and palliation. A male nurse (Bennett 1992a) said:

> I find some of the treatment . . . the medical treatment they receive, um, it's too aggressive, and I question the purpose of it, and is it for them or for the medical research?

Positive Aspects of Caring for People with AIDS

While there are many indications in the data that staff found dealing with death challenging and difficult, there are also indications that respondents learnt and grew from their experiences. Bennett (1992a) notes the following comments by staff. A social worker said:

> . . . It's taught me a lot about how humans grieve, the dignity that they can have when they are dying . . . how people can really come to care for each other, there's a lot of community involvement and community spirit in this disease . . . Human beings tend to hope, even when perhaps it looks like there's nothing left to hope for.

A male nurse comments

> . . . you are helping them die with dignity and feeling you're doing
> something worthwhile.

While staff provide a lot of support for patients, they also receive support in return. Staff often said that they learnt a lot from the patients or that the patients gave them a lot, often in the form of friendship (Bennett 1992a,b). Many described the losses of AIDS as part of a growth process. The positive aspects of AIDS care such as intellectual stimulation, challenge and personal growth were also identified in the research conducted by Horstman and McKusick (1986), Govoni (1988) and Ross and Seeger (1988).

EXPERIENCES OF GRIEF AND COPING STYLES

A number of authors recommend cultivating an internal locus of control to reduce internal stressors associated with care for the dying (Constable and Russell 1986; Martin 1990; Riordan and Saltzer 1992). However, very few studies demonstrate quantifiable data to support this link. The results of research by Bennett and Kelaher (1993a) relate experiences of grief to internal and external coping styles. They revealed that reliance on internal coping strategies and social support was associated with lower levels of grief. In contrast, external coping strategies were associated with higher levels of grief.

These results suggest that staff should be taught coping strategies which involve personal agency rather than relying on external factors to reduce the negative effects of grief. Internal coping is a style that involves staff believing they can make a difference to the situations of their patients. This involves focusing on the contributions that staff make to patient care, rather than a pessimistic focus such as 'no matter what I do, all my patients die'.

Price and Murphy (1984: 49) state that during burnout, the disillusionment and 'resignation to the power of the external environment involves a kind of collapse of the spirit'. This supports the possible links between burnout and external coping styles and suggests that staff need to focus on their ability to make a difference to their patients' lives. Recognition of this may empower staff to view their actions as important and healing, regardless of whether or not they lead to cure.

PRACTICAL IMPLICATIONS AND SUGGESTED INTERVENTIONS

Focus on Psychosocial Successes

Health care professionals need actively to change the focus of care in AIDS from a traditional cure-based approach to a psychosocial achievement model. Working intensively with a dying person is distinctly different from working in areas of health care that focus on cure. There are many examples of AIDS health care that demonstrate psychosocial interventions rather than cure. These include: helping the patient to tell their family about their diagnosis, providing support and facilitating the communication process, helping the patient to decide on the options available such as treatment or palliation, and spending time with the patient when death is approaching.

Shneidman (1978) emphasizes that an important aspect of care is to increase the dying individual's 'psychological comfort' (cited in Clark, 1989). The evaluation measures of effective care must lie in the process of exchange between the professional and the patient and in the 'psychosocial success' in that process. Clark sees these psychosocial successes as distinct from medical or traditional successes. They are defined as those 'identifiable and significant events facilitated by the health care professional which contribute to the emotional well-being of the terminally ill patient and his or her family and friends' (Clark 1989: 119). Clark believes that these successes may act as a partial antidote to burnout. The idea of recounting appears simple and most health care workers can readily recount such instances. The act of recounting assists health care providers to focus on the psychosocial contributions they have made to their clients.

However, few of the psychosocial contributions or successes are documented or even recognized by others. Clark suggests that these successes have been overshadowed by the death of patients. It is the outcome, not the process, that is remembered, and it disallows staff the opportunity of feeling satisfaction at the emotional support and successful interventions they have initiated. Clark suggests a psychosocial success register and formal recognition of these events. This is currently being used by a number of units around the world as part of a research project by Bennett and Kelaher (1993b).

Maintain a Sense of Hope

This is not the traditional view of hoping for a cure, but rather that of carers fostering and maintaining a sense of hope related to the quality of time left and the hope for days or moments that are meaningful and pain-free. Hope is important for patients and staff.

View Grief as an Opportunity for Personal Growth

Once the initial pain of grief has begun to subside, staff may find it possible to view grief and loss as opportunities for growth. Although this is not helpful or beneficial during the intense phases of grief, it may be helpful at a later time. Staff in Bennett's study (1992b) reported episodes of growth and increased appreciation of life following work in the field of HIV/AIDS.

Reduce Internal and External Stressors

Riordan and Saltzer (1992) recommend ways of reducing both external and internal stressors. The reduction of external stressors includes facilitating grieving and closure by providing time to attend funerals and memorials and having weekly support group meetings and supervision with a mentor or counsellor. Also recommended are: creating a staff team approach to work; encouraging open communication between staff and administration; and including staff in decision making when possible. Administrators are further encouraged to arrange proper orientation and ongoing in-service education as well as being aware of the necessary fit between the staff member's personality and the demands of the speciality.

Reduction of internal stressors includes assuming a responsibility for choosing to work with the dying and being aware of personal limitations. Also recommended by Riordan and Saltzer (1992) is a philosophy of involvement which fosters empathic care while maintaining individuality.

Delineate Personal and Professional Lives

In units where staff are caring for ex-lovers and current friends an active attempt needs to be made to separate the duties associated with being a member of staff and those associated with being a friend. While it is difficult for staff to separate care schedules, this needs to be discussed and care plans organized. Staff who are friends should not be the primary care providers, but can visit friends who are patients during short breaks organized specifically for this purpose. Staff need to develop guidelines on how this should be organized and the strategies to use. The roles of friends, lovers and patients need to be delineated and this delineation needs to be discussed with both staff and clients so that all agree to and understand the purpose of separating personal and professional lives. Griffin (1992: 198) does not agree with this idea of delineation and states:

> It is very important to integrate my work . . . as much as possible with my private life, and I do not separate the two . . . sometimes I take them [people with AIDS] home with me . . .

However, Griffin does acknowledge that caregivers need to develop their own style in learning to grieve and grow.

Staff need to be taught self-protection and limiting techniques to reduce the risks associated with overinvolvement with patients. These may involve using time-out techniques in which staff make a conscious effort to do different and new activities that are unrelated to their work. Wessells (1989) states that coping skills and the ability to empathize without merging or fusion are vital. A cognitive separation technique can be incorporated into a relaxation routine. The latter may be beneficial in reducing the anxiety that is associated with high grief levels (Bennett and Kelaher 1993a).

Organize Regular Debriefing Sessions and Support Groups

Debriefing is beneficial to staff and enables opportunities to express and release the volatile emotions discussed in Kavenaugh's stages of adaptation to stress (cited in Price and Murphy 1984). In Bennett and Kelaher's study (1993a), social support was associated with lower levels of intensity of grief, suggesting that discussion groups may diffuse intense emotions and provide support to assist with the adaptation process. A professional mentor or counsellor is useful as a source of guidance and support (Rando 1986, cited in Riordan and Saltzer 1992). Price and Murphy (1984) believe that without deliberate opportunities for staff sharing and mutual support, the burnout rate would almost surely be markedly higher.

CONCLUSION

In conclusion, the experience of grief and loss by carers in AIDS involves experiences of powerlessness, guilt, anxiety, anger, discrimination and despair. Staff who do not adapt or adequately deal with the losses inherent in work in this area may suffer stress and burnout. Staff can be taught strategies to increase their capacity to deal with losses. Focusing on the psychosocial achievements of patient care, promoting a sense of hope, maintaining an internal style of coping, separating personal and professional lives and creating a supportive team approach to care are among the variables that may assist staff with their difficult and demanding roles.

REFERENCES

Baker JM & Kelley LK (1986) Loss: some origins and nursing implications. In DC Longo & RA Williams (eds) *Clinical Practice in Psychosocial Nursing*. Norwalk, CT: Appleton-Century-Crofts pp 75–95

Bennett JA (1987) Nurses talk about the challenge of AIDS *Am J Nursing* **87**: 1150–7

Bennett L (1992a) The impact of HIV/AIDS on health care professionals: psychosocial aspects of care *PhD Thesis* Sydney: Department of Public Health, The University of Sydney

Bennett L (1992b) The experiences of nurses working with hospitalised AIDS patients *Austr J Soc Issues* **27**: 125–43

Bennett L & Kelaher M (1993a) Variables contributing to experiences of grief in HIV/AIDS health care professionals *J Community Psychol* **21**: 210–17

Bennett L & Kelaher M (1993b) Longitudinal determinants of patient care-related stress in HIV/AIDS health professionals *IX Int Con AIDS* (Berlin)

Bennett L, Michie P & Kippax S (1991) Quantitative analysis of burnout and its associated factors in AIDS nursing *AIDS Care* **3**: 181–92

Bolle J (1988) Supporting the deliverers of care: strategies to support nurses and prevent burnout *Nurs Clin North Am* **23**: 843–50

Braybrook T (1993) Coping with grief: communal loss, grieving and bereavement *Austr Fed AIDS Organ Nat AIDS Bull* 7(8): 14–16, Sept

Chapman Dick L (1989) An investigation of the disenfranchised grief of two health care professionals caring for persons with AIDS. In KJ Doka (ed) *Disenfranchised Grief, Recognising Hidden Sorrow* Lexington, MA: Lexington Books pp 55–66

Christ GH & Wiener LS (1985) Psychological issues in AIDS. In VT Devita, S Hellman and SA Rosenberg (eds) *AIDS Etiology: Diagnosis, Treatment and Prevention* Philadelphia PA: Lippincott

Clark EJ (1989) Offsetting burnout in the thanatologic setting: recognition and emphasis of 'psychosocial successes' in social work intervention. In DT Wessells Jr, AH Kutscher, IB Seeland et al (eds) *Professional Burnout in Medicine and the Helping Professions*. New York: The Haworth Press, pp 115–23

Constable J & Russell D (1986) The effects of special support and work environment upon burnout among nurses *J Hum Stress* **12**: 20–6

Doka KJ (1989) (ed) *Disenfranchised Grief, Recognising Hidden Sorrow*. Lexington, MA: Lexington Books

Gordon JH, Ulrich C, Feeley M & Pollack S (1993) Staff distress among haemophilia nurses *AIDS Care* **5**: 359–67

Govoni LA (1988) Psychosocial issues in the care of homosexual men and their significant others *Nurs Clin North Am* **23**: 749–65

Griffin R (1992) Living with AIDS: surviving grief. In P Ahmed (ed) *Living and Dying with AIDS* New York: Plenum Press pp 179–98

Hingley P (1985) Stress in nurse managers *R Coll Nurs Res Soc* June

Horstman W & McKusick L (1986) The impact of AIDS on the physician. In L McKusick (ed) *What to do about AIDS?* Berkeley, CA: University of California Press pp 63–74

Kavenaugh R (1973) *Facing Death* Los Angeles: Nash Publishing

Maj M (1991) Psychological problems of families and health care workers dealing with people infected with human immunodeficiency virus 1 *Acta Psychiatr Scand* **83**: 161–8

Martin DA (1990) Effects of ethical dilemmas on stress felt by nurses providing care to AIDS patients *Crit Care Nurs Q* **12**(4): 53–62

Miller D (1988) HIV and social psychiatry *Br Med Bull* **44**: 130–48

Morin SF & Batchelor WF (1984) Responding to the psychological crisis of AIDS *Public Health Rep* **99**: 4–9

Nash A (1985) Bereavement: staff support *Nursing* **2**: 1288

Piemme JA & Bolle JL (1990) Coping with grief in response to caring for persons with AIDS *Am J Occup Ther* **44**: 266–9

Price T & Bergen B (1977) The relationship of death as a source of stress for nurses on a coronary care unit *Omega* **8**: 229–38

Price DM & Murphy PA (1984) Staff burnout in the perspective of grief theory *Death Educ* **8**: 47–58

Rando T (1986) *Loss and Anticipatory Grief* Lexington MA: Lexington Books

Riordon RJ & Saltzer SK (1992) Burnout prevention among health care providers working with the terminally ill: a review of the literature *Omega* **25**: 17–24

Ross M & Seeger V (1988) Determinants of reported burnout in health professionals associated with the care of patients with AIDS *AIDS* **2**: 395–7

Shneidman ES (1978) Some aspects of psychotherapy with dying patients. In CA Garfield (ed) *Psychosocial Care of the Dying Patient* New York: McGraw-Hill

Shulman LC & Mantell JE (1988) The AIDS crisis: a United States health care perspective *Soc Sci Med* **26**: 979–88

Stroebe W & Stroebe MS (1987) *Bereavement and Health: The Psychological and Physical Consequences of Partner Loss* New York: Cambridge University Press

Wessells DT Jr (1989) The etiology of job stress. In DT Wessels Jr, AH Kutscher, IB Seeland et al (eds) *Professional Burnout in Medicine and the Helping Professions* New York: The Haworth Press

Wolcott DL, Fawzy FI & Pasnau RO (1985) Acquired immune deficiency syndrome (AIDS) and consultation liaison psychiatry *Gen Hosp Psychiatry* **7**: 280–92

CHAPTER 7

Allowing Someone To Die

Calliope C. S. Farsides

University of Keele, UK

MEDICAL AND ETHICAL MODELS OF CARE

The medical model of care in its simplest form almost inevitably regards death as a sign of failure. In fact, in the case of the terminally ill, failure may have been admitted some considerable time prior to death, when the type of treatment offered of necessity shifted from curative to palliative. Despite clear evidence to the contrary, a terminal prognosis may be accompanied by the belief that 'there is nothing more to be done'. This places significant burdens on those who choose to care for people with incurable diseases and a terminal prognosis, as the ultimate form of success is never available to them, and the profoundest failure is inevitable at some point in the future.

The person with AIDS poses particular problems for the crudely medical perspective, as she does not as yet experience a phase during which the illness is seen as curable in the sense that the virus can be destroyed. Of course, much can be done to treat the opportunistic infections and diseases s/he may suffer from, and carers can, and do, make conscious efforts to prolong life. However, in the AIDS context, the type of care offered has to go far beyond that dictated by purely medical needs, and the idea of what is good for the patient may need to be radically reinterpreted. Part of securing the good of the patient will necessarily involve addressing issues concerning his/her almost inevitably premature death.

In this chapter it will be suggested that carers may be helped to fulfil this task by helping them to understand that there are ethical justifications for questioning the medical model's preoccupation with life-prolonging treatment. One's moral duties to a patient can, on occasions, have as much to do with securing the type of death they desire as with helping them

Grief and AIDS. Edited by L. Sherr.
©1995 John Wiley & Sons Ltd.

to live. By discussing the ethical issues surrounding death and dying, and rehearsing the arguments supporting non-treatment, withdrawal of treatment, or maybe even death-hastening treatments, teams of carers can be prepared to help the patient who welcomes death as effectively as those who cherish life.

This would be valuable, as there may come a point at which the patient and/or the carers begin to question whether good reasons remain for pursuing the medical treatments that are available. This thought might relate in turn to thoughts about whether the patient's life is any longer 'a life worth living'. It is possible that some will reach a stage in their illness where the dominant image of death as the great evil might, in fact, be replaced by that of death as the liberating friend. Thus they might come to question the basic assumption that more life is better than less, and believe instead that their life should end sooner rather than later.

If and when this point is reached it is important for the carer to realize that they still have a part to play. Their skills do not become redundant once death is a desired or accepted outcome. Now, however, their role may be concerned with permitting or facilitating a good death, as opposed to helping the person within their care to live, and this may be a task for which their training leaves them less than fully equipped.

It could be argued that time spent on ethical reflection and discussion would be time well spent, even in the busiest of units. Sharing moral perspectives, and rehearsing potential conflicts or dilemmas, would allow carers to prepare for the time when they can (or should) do little more to sustain a person's body, but can still do much to protect their dignity and autonomy. Increasingly, professionals seek out opportunities to clarify their own moral position through formal courses in ethics, but a simple discussion over coffee once a week can also make a difference. This chapter delves quite heavily into theoretical issues, but hopefully in such a way as to facilitate coffee-break discussions.

QUALITY VERSUS QUANTITY OF LIFE

The concept of a 'life worth living' is one which is employed both at the beginning and at the end of life, by those who feel that quality of life considerations are crucial to any decision about whether life should be terminated or prolonged. Thus, reference may be made to the predicted quality of life of a handicapped foetus in deciding whether or not to terminate a pregnancy (Kuhse and Singer 1985). Similarly, the degree of brain damage suffered by a traffic accident victim may be assessed prior to engaging full life-support systems. It is not an unproblematic concept, and there are those who reject it completely, preferring to maintain that all life is sacred irrespective of its quality (Glover 1988; Kuhse 1987).

Some of those who believe in 'the sanctity of life' go on to attack any proposal which has as its direct intention the cessation or foreshortening of life, unless the life in question fails to qualify for the description 'innocent'. Thus they might accept and indeed advocate capital punishment, whilst vociferously campaigning against abortion and active euthanasia.

Others will be prepared to say that at a certain point the quality of life becomes important, maybe even decisive, in determining whether that life should continue (Harris 1985), but there may not be easy agreement concerning the point at which this is so. People will disagree as to what level of handicap provides a justification for the abortion of a foetus, or what level of suffering permits mention of euthanasia. Furthermore, there could be dispute concerning who is entitled to decide that a person's life is not worth living; is it a decision that can justifiably be made by anyone other than the person in question (Buchanen and Brock 1989)?

INDIVIDUAL CHOICE AND PROXY DECISION MAKING

The 'simplest' case a carer might meet is where an individual has prepared an advance directive, as discussed in Chapter 9, and although near to death is sufficiently competent to endorse the provisions therein. This situation would allow the patient to evaluate their own condition, and judge whether they felt that life really was 'not worth living', precisely in the way they had predicted when preparing their living will. The choice could be viewed as voluntary and autonomous, and the carer could therefore decide that they had a duty to respect it.

In such a situation some responsibility rests with the carer to explore the reasons behind the request being made, even if they have been previously stated in the terms discussed here. It is important, for example, to ascertain that the patient is not choosing to give up on life merely because they feel themselves to be a burden to those around them. If the patient feels that their life in terms of its quality is still worth living, the carers must demonstrate that the 'burden' of caring is willingly borne, and that death would be unnecessary self-sacrifice.

A less clear-cut case than that cited above occurs when a document expressing the patient's wishes exists, but the patient is no longer competent to judge whether this is the point at which to activate it. For example, a person with AIDS might be motivated to prepare an advanced directive because of the fear of dementia. If such dementia does strike, the person will no longer be capable of endorsing the provisions of the document. Here partners, families, friends and carers may have to decide whether or not to abide by the previously stated wishes of the patient, taking upon themselves the responsibility of confirming the fact that her life is no longer worth living. This might be particularly difficult where those involved hold strongly opposing views as to whether or not life is sacred, and whether or when quality should be allowed to count.

Problems can also arise when caring for children with life-threatening or terminal diseases. Here the issue of competence takes on a different guise, and a decision may have to be made about how much control, if any, the child should be allowed over treatment or non-treatment decisions (Freeman and McDonnell 1987: 57–62). If it is decided that the child is not sufficiently competent to determine if and when her life ceases to be worth living, a burdensome responsibility falls on the parents, as the most obvious proxies, to decide what is in their child's best interest. It is at least possible that parents who decide that the death of their child is the preferred outcome will meet resistance from carers unable to cope with so premature a death, and thus so substantial a 'failure'. If, as may sometimes be the case in AIDS medicine, the parents have predeceased the child, non-related carers may have to become particularly closely involved in decisions that they find difficult to face.

One way or another, in cases such as these the carers' involvement is morally more demanding, and those who wish to give any consideration to the question of euthanasia generally feel happier with voluntary requests than with cases involving some degree of proxy consent. In practical terms there may be much to be said for raising and discussing the issue of the manner in which a person hopes to die long before their death is imminent, precisely so that they can be afforded the opportunity to decide what control, if any, they wish to exercise over their death. It would then be advisable to share the fruits of such discussions with those most likely to be placed in the position of proxy should the individual lose competence before death.

Let us now assume for the sake of argument that some carers will encounter patients who have decided that they no longer wish to carry on living, and who are in a position to make these wishes known. Let us also assume that, while eschewing a strong 'sanctity of life' position, the carer feels that their duty of care is ordinarily understandable as a duty to protect and promote life.

RESPECTING A PATIENT'S WISH TO DIE

Realistically there are very few practitioners who interpret the professional duty to care as analogous to a clear-cut duty to prolong life *irrespective* of its quality or of the patient's wishes (BMA 1993: 147–77). None the less, given the professional and cultural emphasis placed on the notion of curing and treating, and the prevailing attitudes towards death, it could be very difficult for some carers to accede even to a clear request not to treat if they know it would inevitably hasten the death. This would be especially true if, in their opinion, the person's life was still of a quality they themselves would consider acceptable. In some cases the carer might continue to feel that their professional duty demands that they intervene further and continue to treat.

In such cases, a moral argument might be required that shows them that they have fulfilled their professional (and moral) duty to the patient even if they decide that they will do no more to prolong or preserve life. Such an argument exists in the form of the distinction made within moral philosophy between ordinary and extraordinary means.

Ordinary and Extraordinary Means

This formal distinction was originally employed within Roman Catholic doctrine to allow a practical distinction to be made between the refusal of some forms of medical intervention and suicide, the latter being a sin (Beauchamp and Childress 1989: 151–4). In its most famous form the distinction holds that while a person has a duty not to refuse all 'ordinary' forms of care, they can in certain circumstances refuse 'extraordinary' forms, even where these are potentially life-prolonging. More useful for our purposes is a permissible reformulation which allows that whilst a carer has a duty to provide (and a patient has an accompanying duty to accept) all 'ordinary' forms of treatment, the carer can withhold (and the patient refuse) those forms of treatment deemed to be 'extraordinary'.

When it comes to deciding which treatments are 'ordinary' and which are 'extraordinary' it is important not to translate the latter to 'unusual' or 'strange'; rather, they are taken to be 'all medicines, treatments, and operations, which cannot be obtained or used without excessive expense, pain or other inconvenience, or which, if used would not offer a reasonable hope of benefit' (Kelly 1951: 550). Conversely, 'ordinary means are all medicines, treatments and operations, which offer a reasonable hope of benefit and which can be obtained and used without excessive expense, pain, or other inconvenience' (Kelly 1951: 550).

In formulating the doctrine, particular care was taken not to refer explicitly to the quality of life of the patient, but one cannot fail to import the idea into one's evaluations of treatments vis-à-vis the burden they impose, which is essentially the issue at stake. In a near-death situation with a desperately ill patient the burden of a particular treatment may be much heavier than if the same treatment were administered to someone in a stronger state. One young physician gave the following account of the moment in which she realized this truth.

> He asked for more help. I stuck a plastic cannula into his nose to give him some more oxygen. I gave him potassium in his IV line. I told him his problems were being corrected and we would discuss chemotherapy options in the morning. After I left the hospital that night, feeling exhausted but confident I'd given 'my all', another physician on duty was called to see my patient. Raphael asked the physician to help him. The physician stopped the intravenous fluid and potassium, cancelled the blood testing and the transfusion, and simply gave Raphael some morphine. I was told Raphael smiled and thanked the doctor for helping him and then expired later that evening. (Scannell 1988: 103–4)

It was surely *because* of the hopelessness of Raphael's situation and the imminence of his death that otherwise routine procedures became, if not cruel, then at least burdensome. None the less, the doctrine does allow the carer to ask 'what burden the treatment?' if they cannot face the question 'what value the life?' That is to say, the emphasis is placed on the question of what price the patient has to bear, rather than whether the patient is in any sense worth saving.

So, the first available option supported by ethical argument is for the carer to decide that, whilst treatments are available, the cost attached is too high given the small benefit on offer, so the treatment should not be given. If treatments are already under way which become burdensome with the patient's worsening condition they could be withdrawn.

However, once again the person with AIDS offers us a particular challenge. In the original formulation, a strict limitation is traditionally placed upon the contexts within which the doctrine can be employed by stating that the patient must be suffering from a terminal disease, and death must be imminent. In the case of a person with AIDS-related illness it is possible that they will decide that their life is no longer worth living, not because of the severity of a condition from which they are suffering at any one time, but rather because of the increasing frequency with which they are struck by opportunistic infections and debilitating body changes. The oscillating disease process provides a quite different context within which to decide whether life remains worth living, or treatments remain worth giving. For example, an individual who suffers from a third bout of pneumonia in nine months might question the worth of his/her continued existence, even though the condition could be treated and the current illness does not necessarily place the patient in the terminal phase of care. Many would respond to this example by suggesting that adequate counselling and support will allow a patient to cope with increasing bouts of illness, but nevertheless one should appreciate that some people will feel that life is no longer worth living once it is characterized by illness and repeated courses of treatment, even if they can still enjoy intermittent periods of relatively good health.

Examples such as these pose problems for the distinction between ordinary and extraordinary means, first because it moves our considerations away from a classic near-death situation, and secondly because it opens the possibility of a patient wishing to refuse treatment which is in no sense extraordinary. This leads to the question of whether it is ever morally justifiable to withhold or withdraw treatments that have a good chance of helping the patient, and that are not burdensome in the sense described above. In response to this question the philosopher could choose to introduce another distinction, which is that made between an act and an omission.

Acts and Omissions Doctrine

It is intuitively accepted by many people that it is far worse to act in such a way as to make something bad happen than it is to fail to act, even when this results in the same bad thing happening. So, to use a lurid example, it is far worse to send rotten food parcels to starving people in Africa than it is to fail to give money to Oxfam, even though the result is the same in both cases, i.e. people die of poisoning or starvation (Foot 1978). This translates in philosophical terms into the Acts and Omissions Distinction, and this distinction in turn lies behind that between active and passive euthanasia.

To return to the example cited above in which one fails to give a patient quite standard treatment for a treatable condition, it could be argued that by omitting to treat him/her (assuming this is his/her wish) one is not responsible for her death in the way that one would be if one did something to make him/her die. However, this assumption might be questioned on two counts. First, one could ask whether a conscious decision not to treat is sufficiently passive to count as an omission rather than an action – this is a rather theoretical point which can be ignored on this occasion. One should not refrain, however, from raising a second question: is it really the case that *'actions* that result in some bad consequence are always worse than *failures to act* that have the same consequence' (McNaughton 1989) (assuming only for the sake of argument that death is always a 'bad consequence')?

Consider the following example. Claire has been HIV-positive for six years, and was given an AIDS diagnosis two years ago. She is now desperately ill and close to death, her pain is uncontrollable and her dignity is slowly ebbing away. Despite the best efforts of her carers, and the loving attention of family and friends, she herself wishes to die. She is not being treated by any 'extraordinary means', so there is no treatment that can be withdrawn under that justification. She agrees with her carers that no further steps will be taken to treat her condition should a need arise, she will be kept comfortable, and will not be resuscitated if she stops breathing. What she really wants is for someone to help her to die *now*.

Some people will be prepared to ask whether, setting aside the legal issues, it would really be worse to *actively* bring about her death at a suitably appointed time (Rachels 1975). Having agreed not to treat her, her carers have joined in her intention that she should die sooner rather than later. The motives of all those involved are pure, and all that any further time will buy her is further suffering. In such a case, some philosophers would argue that it would be preferable actively to kill her than passively to allow her to die, yet the acts and omissions doctrine ensures a prohibition on active intervention. In practice the distinction is usually invoked to claim that killing a person is never justifiable, even if allowing them to die may sometimes be so (Beauchamp and Childress 1989: 138–47).

It is highly likely that carers will feel that *acting* to bring about a person's death is different in some important respects to *allowing* them to die. The question is whether the difference is in any way interesting or significant at a moral level. There are various arguments one could provide to support the distinction at this point, but one might none the less conclude that, in certain situations where the appropriate people have agreed that death is the desired outcome, it is more humane to ensure that death happens quickly and easily, as opposed to trusting that an opportunity not to treat will naturally arise. If this is the case one might want to find out if there is any way of getting around the prohibition on direct action, whilst remaining within the appropriate moral (and legal) boundaries.

Carers may attempt to do so with the assistance of another philosophical doctrine, but it will be shown that this is only really possible given a few sleights of hand. The doctrine in question is a complex one, once again born of Roman Catholic preoccupations, and it is known as the doctrine of double effect.

The Doctrine of Double Effect

Basically the doctrine of double effect states that 'there is a morally relevant difference between the intended effects of a person's action and the non-intended though foreseen effects of the action' (Beauchamp and Childress 1989: 127). Those who employ the doctrine believe that one is never allowed directly to form the intention to do something bad, even if it would bring about a significantly greater good, that is, they reject the idea of the end justifying the means. In this context, they would define killing as an evil, and therefore claim that direct killing is prohibited, even in the name of ending severe suffering.

However, one might be permitted to pursue a morally good end even if something bad (i.e. death) was a foreseen and unavoidable side-effect of doing so. So, for example, were one to be primarily concerned with controlling a person's pain, one could administer increasingly high doses of certain drugs, even though one knew that these would eventually cause the person to die. Returning to the previously cited example of Raphael, the morphine given to control his pain could be an example of this type.

To be true to the doctrine one would have to be sure that if other drugs were available which did not hasten death they would be used. Similarly, a carer would have to show that they in no way directly intended, as part of what they were doing, to hasten death. The aim has to be the relief of pain and suffering, and death can only be accepted as a side-effect (albeit foreseeable) of achieving this aim. If Raphael's physician intended to speed up his death by administering the morphine the example would not fall under the doctrine of double effect.

This is the theory; in practice the doctrine is often implicitly referred to in situations where there is in fact a clear, shared intention to facilitate death, that is, a clear intention to use drugs precisely *because* they will hasten death is presented as a non-controversial treatment decision. This is not honest dealing, but it may be all that is available to the carer who wants to assist in a good death through action rather than inaction, and remain free from the threat of prosecution.

RETURNING TO THE PRACTICALITIES

The distinctions and justifications discussed in this chapter are largely utilized by philosophers who hold to the idea that lives should be preserved and killing is intrinsically wrong. As such they fit more readily with the medical model of care than some other moral perspectives on death and dying. Furthermore, they are available for use by those who do not as yet wish to endorse active forms of euthanasia. However, they do allow a carer and patient to decide together that death should occur sooner rather than later and, albeit by omission rather than action, they provide the moral justification for exerting some control over the natural course of events.

Discussing the ways in which morality allows us to facilitate a patient's dying should help carers to feel comfortable with the idea that the death of a patient is not in and of itself a sign of failure. How and when the patient dies is relevant to whether the death is a good death, and a good death is the penultimate stage of successful care.

Coming to terms with this fact could spare the carer from the burden of thinking 'I should have done more'. The ethical arguments presented here might instead lead carers to acknowledge that (in treatment terms) they could, and should, have done less for some patients. It is possible to fulfil one's duty of care by respecting the autonomy of the patient, preventing avoidable suffering, and allowing the patient to decide if and when their life is no longer worth prolonging.

Some individuals will make this decision for themselves, without involving their carers, and if they have the means and the will to do so they may choose suicide. This is a complex moral issue in its own right (Glover 1988: 170–9), but it might be worth mentioning in this context that a willingness on the part of carers to be involved in the death of their patients could spare some individuals from the lonely act of suicide, and also spare the bereaved some of the particular problems associated with that type of death.

If they feel comfortable with the idea of facilitating death the carer will in turn be better able to fulfil the final duty of care to their patient, which is to facilitate the grieving of those who have been left behind. If carers allow themselves to understand that death was an outcome chosen by their patient, and secured with their support, they can help the bereaved unhindered by the guilt associated with failure. To do this they have to acknowledge openly that they have taken part in the patient's death in preference to prolonging their life.

In future years 'taking part' might mean administering a lethal injection; at present it can go no further than standing back and allowing someone to die, or knowingly treating their pain or distress in such a way as to make death unavoidable. However, even these limited forms of involvement allow carers the opportunity to interpret death in a newly positive light as a part of a process over which they and the patient can exercise some control, and for which they should not be afraid to take responsibility.

REFERENCES

Beauchamp TL & Childress JF (1989) *Principles of Biomedical Ethics* Oxford: Oxford University Press

BMA Ethics Science and Information Division (1993) *Medical Ethics Today: Its Practice and Philosophy* London: BMJ Publishing Group

Buchanen AE & Brock DW (1989) *Deciding For Others* Cambridge: Cambridge University Press

Foot P (1978) Euthanasia. In *Virtues and Vices* Oxford: Blackwell pp 19–32

Freeman J & McDonnell K (1987) *Tough Decisions* Oxford: Oxford University Press

Glover J (1988) *Causing Death and Saving Lives* Harmondsworth: Penguin

Harris J (1985) *The Value of Life* London: Routledge

Kelly G (1951) The duty to preserve life *Theol Stud* **12**: 550

Kuhse H (1987) *The Sanctity of Life Doctrine in Medicine: A Critique* Oxford: Clarendon Press

Kuhse H & Singer P (1985) *Should the Baby Live?* Oxford: Oxford University Press

McNaughton D (1989) Killing and letting die. In P de Cruz & D McNaughton (eds) *By What Right?* Newcastle-under-Lyme, Staffordshire: Penrhos Publications

Rachels J (1975) Active and passive euthanasia *N Eng J Med* **292**: 78–80

Scannell K (1988) Skills and pills. In I Rieder & P Rupplet (eds) *AIDS: The Women* Pittsburgh, PA: Cleis Press

CHAPTER 8

Crisis of the Psyche: Psychotherapeutic Considerations on AIDS, Loss and Hope

S. Christopher W. Mead

Rijksuniversiteit, Leiden, The Netherlands

and

Hessel W. A. Willemsen

Rijksuniversiteit, Leiden, The Netherlands

There is, specifically, much about AIDS that forces us to confront loss, abandonment and death that all of us in the Western world – gay, straight, male, female, the economically advantaged, disadvantaged, racially and ethnically oppressed – have felt ourselves so immune from disfiguring illness, from early death . . . AIDS has meant coming to terms with limitations, with a finitude we had thought we might evade. (Downing 1989: 280)

During the past decade much has been and still needs to be said about HIV/AIDS, loss and grief. To date, our knowledge in the field of HIV/AIDS about the impact of disease upon the individual psyche of the patient and the emotional support systems comes from work with other life-threatening diseases such as cancer, as well as from quantitative research in the area of coping and adaptation, health-related quality of life and from limited qualitative and phenomenological research concerning patients. The research in the field is impressive and informative, yet, health care professionals and psychotherapists are frequently left longing for ways of understanding this disease that would

Grief and AIDS. Edited by L. Sherr.
©1995 John Wiley & Sons Ltd.

help them to understand the lived human experience and to liberate themselves and their patients from prevalent limiting psychological models in working with this disease and with these populations.

Patients, friends and colleagues remain our most important teachers in this area of work. Additionally, there is much to be learned from the AIDS poets such as Klein (1989), novelists and AIDS biographers such as Monette (1988) and political essayists such as Sontag (1988), all of whom help to illuminate images and metaphors that give us insight and entrance to exploring other ways of living and deepening human experience. They teach us about liberation of the psyche from traditional models and help us to unlock emotions and to re-orient experience, all of which can help individuals to come to terms with this disease, as well as contribute to a sense of hope and release from despair.

In this pandemic, many have been left behind by the death of loved ones. The impact upon human lives on a micro and macro level, on a personal and community level, is enormous. HIV is having a devastating effect upon our planet and its people. It decimates communities and can destroy a whole generation of young people, not because of war, but instead because of something as beautiful and simple and basic as one human being loving another. Concerns on this level engender fear and anger. Human beings remain reckless and may overlook the possibility that the human race is still vulnerable to destruction, disease and illness even though medical science seemed to have conquered such diseases as smallpox and polio and deluded us that we could live for ever. It is a saddening and disconcerting judgement on our society that so many psychotherapy patients say: 'HIV disease is the best thing that has happened to me in my life'. There is an anxiety about forgetting those who were loved and about losing still more.

HIV/AIDS can be viewed from various perspectives: psychological, political, sociological and biological. It can also be studied in the major thematic areas that emerge from the literature: at-risk populations, clinical settings, disease progression and impact. However, no matter how one examines the scope of HIV infection, the one theme that transcends the literature is the issue of loss. HIV infection and AIDS encompass not only the process of dying, but also a constant process of loss, which includes adaptation and coping with change on behavioural, physical, emotional and intrapsychic levels. HIV/AIDS patients struggle with great uncertainty about their illness, their treatment and their future. Most HIV patients are young adults in the most productive years of life. These people must confront and cope with many losses throughout their illness. They must confront the losses of physical strength and attractiveness, the loss of previous sexual behaviours and intimate relationships, the possible loss of employment and employability, loss of hopes and plans for the future and the loss of friends, lovers and family as well as the loss of self-esteem; their self-image is severely damaged or even lost. Additionally, they must deal with the possibility of the loss of mental functioning due to neuro-psychiatric complications and AIDS dementia complex, multiple losses within the community and the loss of the possibility of a cure (Solomon and Mead 1987; Macks 1989; Winiarski 1991). Perhaps the most important and difficult loss that confronts the HIV/AIDS patient is that of meaningfulness in life as they have known it. The individual must accept that a change has occurred in their external world and that they are required to make a corresponding change in their internal, representational world and to reorganize, readjust and perhaps to reorient their behaviour (Freud 1960) and attitudes so that they are in alignment with life's present possibilities. Indeed, HIV infection is a disease of loss.

REVIEW OF THE LITERATURE

An enormous amount has been written on HIV/AIDS and loss, coping and adaptation during the past decade. Much contemporary psychological literature is critical of the shortcomings of the traditional grief models; it neglects the more complicated psychological, social and political issues that emerge with HIV/AIDS grief and loss (Geis, Fuller and Rush 1986; Macks 1989; O'Neil 1989; Schoen and Schindelman 1989; Schwartzenberg 1992).

Confronted by the threat of death, AIDS patients experience feelings of grief similar to those of all people experiencing catastrophic or chronic illness and loss, though the characteristics of this disease are obviously different: political issues, economic and social stigma, homophobia, fear of contracting the disease or of being a carrier, prostitution, drug abuse and sexuality are only a few of the concerns that complicate HIV/AIDS grief (Geis, Fuller and Rush 1986; Klein and Fletcher 1986; Macks 1989). Because the issues are complicated, new grief models have been developed (Biller and Rice 1990) and old models (Kubler-Ross 1969) have been reexamined and modified (Dane 1991) to include the compounding factors related to multiple loss of persons with AIDS (see Chapter 1 by Lorraine Sherr). O'Neil (1989) discusses the tasks of grief in the light of early attachment theory as expounded by Bowlby (1981) and Worden (1982), as well as the risk of internalized homophobia and the absence of institutional recognition of same-sex relationships.

Clinicians need to differentiate AIDS-related grief from other types of loss. O'Neil mentions the adverse effects of multiple, cumulative loss and the importance of finding meaning in ongoing adversity.

Both Schwartzenberg (1992) and Saynor (1988) discuss issues specifically related to the homosexual community and the unselfish demonstration of support.

The HIV/AIDS patient and the survivors deal with difficult and complicated tasks. Worden (1991) highlights lack of social support as well as issues of contagion, untimely deaths, protracted illness, disfigurement and neurological complications and how these factors influence the grieving behaviour of the survivors. The literature describes different psychotherapeutic perspectives that may be helpful in dealing with increasing dependency due to illness and loss. The most frequently mentioned psychotherapeutic techniques include: crisis intervention, supportive treatment, cognitive–behavioural, existential and psycho-analytical oriented therapies.

In the psychoanalytic and analytic schools of thought there is little discussion in the literature of HIV/AIDS issues and the psyche, conscious and unconscious phenomena. The literature that is available is primarily concerned with case studies. Some studies (Ramos 1989; Hildebrand 1992) concern homosexual men in analysis; they seem to focus primarily upon how the patient's homosexual 'pathology' is acted out with their HIV/AIDS and in their analysis. A few articles address the role of homophobia from a psychoanalytic perspective (Moss 1992) as well as some of the psychoanalytic issues raised in working with HIV/AIDS patients, such as the therapeutic parameters and trust (Sadowey 1991; Blencher 1993).

Freud (1917) and Lindemann (1944) both discuss the issue of loss as object loss. The image of the grieving individual presented by Freud is that of a social isolate who, unaided by friends and family, withdraws from the outside world to work through a painful process of detachment from the beloved who has died. Freud's idea that 'working through' grief and loss is essential for a successful outcome to bereavement has had a persisting influence on subsequent theories and therapeutic approaches. Wilson (1988) and Meyers (1987) discuss Kleinian object-relations theory and the relevance to HIV/AIDS treatment.

Like Freud, Bowlby (1971, 1975, 1981) and O'Neil (1989) view grief as the emotional response to the disruption of the bereaved and the loss of the primary attachment figure. Bowlby's attachment theory discusses grief and loss in terms of an instinct metaphor borrowed from ethnology. One of the implications of this theory is that the impact of loss and concomitant emotions can be lessened by forming substitute attachments.

From a Jungian analytical psychology perspective there are only a few publications. Bosnak (1989) and Wilmer (1991) both wrote on dreams and the individuation process of a person dying of AIDS. Bosnak describes his own countertransference reaction to his patient's increasing dependency, loss and dying and the intrapsychic process, and the manner in which his personal reaction facilitated the analytical process and the patient's individuation process.

It appears that most Freudian and Jungian analysts focus their analysis upon the dying process itself and treat HIV/AIDS and loss as they would any other chronic illness or disease that may eventually lead to death. Such a process is understandable. However, it strengthens the analytical bias that places almost the entire emphasis upon the individual psyche in the consulting room and neglects the socio-political world. As HIV infection has revolutionized modern medicine and the patient–physician relationship, it may also force analysts to re-examine their own biases and allow for a fuller contextual analysis that includes the socio-political environment.

Most of the present HIV/AIDS literature focuses upon coping and adaptation, in which the cognitive–behavioural perspective dominates. The coping model of Cohen and Lazarus (1973) is frequently quoted in the research on HIV/AIDS loss and grief. They present five types of coping strategies: direct action, inhibition of action, intrapsychic processes, information-seeking and turning to others for support. Direct action and a fighting spirit leading to a dynamic personal development and inhibition of action, as a cause of homophobia, are described, for example, by Mansson (1992). The importance of turning to others for support and information-seeking is scattered throughout much of the literature in the form of support, information and education groups as well as its role in individual, relational and family psychotherapy (Solomon and Mead 1987; Dilly, Pies and Helquist 1989; Winiarski 1991).

The cognitive–behavioural tradition so prevalent and facilitating in coping and adapting to HIV/AIDS is heavily focused upon the idea of learned helplessness (Seligman 1975). For example, when an animal or person is faced with an outcome that is independent of his/her responses, s/he learns that his/her response is ineffectual and helpless in affecting the outcome of his/her life. A person grieving a loss will have many feelings of loss of control and the approach to understanding grief and loss offered by this model, even though effective in education and coping, remains limited. Exercising self-control, for example, is believed to be one of the most important interventions: perceptions of personal control were associated with better adjustment to AIDS (Taylor et al 1991). However, the model cannot account for complicated pathology and such issues as delay or even absence of grief.

The existential impact of AIDS and HIV on a person's life is enormous. This population must live with dying and great uncertainty. The lived experience of coping with HIV disease unfolds from the initial diagnosis of being HIV-seropositive through the diagnosis of AIDS and eventual death. McCain and Gramling (1992) describe the disease in terms of the following processes: living with dying, fighting the sickness and getting worn out.

The majority of this population are members of larger communities where AIDS, death and dying are omnipresent; many have preceded them in their death and many will follow. Writers and existential philosophers such as Tillich (1955), May (1953, 1969), May, Angel and Ellenberger (1958) and Yalom (1980) are frequently referenced in the literature because they describe the importance of framing many issues in existential terms. Death, loss and alienation, as many philosophers have proposed, are at the heart of the existential anxiety. Such existential issues as fear of loss or fear of intimacy are observed phenomena in many HIV/ AIDS patients. Issues of abandonment, quality of life, suicide and euthanasia are present at some point and to some degree with every HIV/ AIDS person (Winiarski 1991).

NORMAL PSYCHOLOGICAL DEVELOPMENT

HIV/AIDS loss is a crisis of the psyche. Seventy per cent of HIV/AIDS patients are between the ages of 20 and 39 years old (Macks 1989). These individuals are being robbed of their normal psychological development and are being required to take on the developmental tasks of old age. Young people, especially those who had not previously mastered major life crises, losses or serious illnesses, may lack the experience to cope with the issues they now face.

The purpose of the first half of life is different from that of the second half of life. Normal psychological development requires that the person leave home and develop a sense of 'I', an ego. The first half of life is about the experience of separateness and identity, becoming independent of parents, developing meaningful relationships, learning about the world, gaining status in society through work, and learning how to enjoy and create a meaningful life. In the second half of life, there is a gradual decline of the aims and goals of the first half and a movement toward the preparation for death. This period of time is about letting go, reflection, awareness and acceptance of the choices and limitations of one's own life as it was lived and about passing onto the next generation the experience and the wisdom acquired (Jung 1956, 1960; Gordon 1978, 1993; Baker & Wheelwright 1982). This process requires a reversal of the values that were necessary during the first half of life.

In normal development a change in attitude begins at mid-life, around 35 or 40 years old. This mid-life crisis is the crisis of the unlived life of the first 35 or 40 years. Jung (1966) addresses this issue in *Two Essays in Analytical Psychology*. He says, 'the problems that crop up at this age are no longer to be solved by the old recipes: the hand of the clock cannot be put back. What youth found and must find outside, the man [or woman] of life's afternoon must find within himself [or herself]' (Jung 1966: 75). Any crisis, such as the death of a loved one, serious illness or even unexpected success, can stimulate the psyche and disturb the balance. Crisis brings with it the possibility of psychological growth as well as the possibility of destruction. New solutions are needed, in fact demanded, and if not found there is the dangerous risk of reconstituting in old ways. Normal development carries with it generally accepted life events and crises, some of which are biological and some cultural: separating from mother, first day in school, adolescence, dating, marriage, career, death of parents, children growing up, retirement, old age and death. It may also include divorce and remarriage. Crises usually involve events associated with loss and a subjective experience associated with a break in previous attachments to persons, places or things. Alternatively, they involve situations that disrupt the customary modes of behaviour, circumstances and plans for the future. Crises present the individual with the opportunity to question and re-evaluate many previously held assumptions and values and to replace them with others that are more in line with reality as it is currently experienced and lived. New meaning may or may not be found (Liberman 1975; Zinkin 1989). Crises bring with them a breaking up of the personality, allowing for the possible emergence of new patterns. They offer the opportunity for a second chance to do correctly what was not completed earlier.

In the many crises of HIV/AIDS the person's subjective feelings of control and loss are elicited. Living with this disease for the individual and his/her support system can lead to a loss and break in previous attachments to persons, places and things. It may also reactivate dormant conflicts and an individual's ambivalent feelings about their own sexuality, drug abuse or prostitution. If the person's inner attitudes are not secure and their self-esteem is closely tied to matching cultural norms, the individual is particularly vulnerable to societal attitudes.

Crises are experienced as a danger to the psyche. During times of acute crisis or feelings of loss the patient may resort to old solutions that are no longer appropriate in the present state of illness. Loss and pain must be accepted. However, owing to their magnitude they may throw the psyche out of balance. Hopefully, the person does not resort to old ways of dealing with situations or fall back into regressive complexes but instead can look toward a more creative and yet unknown solution in the unconscious. By attending to dreams and images, by listening to those far-away voices and making them more conscious and by staying with the dualities of a conflict a compensatory meaning may be found and a bridge toward a higher level of knowledge, awareness and acceptance achieved.

A phenomenon observed in psychotherapy practice with HIV/AIDS patients is that some patients appear to have an accelerated movement towards individuation and wholeness while others live their illness with little psychological growth or development. There is nothing beautiful or romantic about HIV infection. It is an ugly and devastating disease. As can be very easily understood, some people experience their illness as a thief, robber or rapist. Perhaps it is the fear of death that fights against change. To accept change means to accept linear time (past, present and future) and this brings with it an awareness of an inevitable end. Accepting death means inevitable confrontation with non-existence, an awareness that brings with it pain and challenge.

This is probably what Gordon (1993) describes when she talks of the wholeness–separation axis. If a person has invested most of their emotional life in the experience of separateness and identity – the ego and its functions – they will regard death as the enemy, for it will take all that has been valued. On the other hand, the person whose emotional needs are primarily directed toward synthesis and wholeness may be able to look upon death with a sense of completion, a life that has been lived with both its blessings and curses.

Observations in work with HIV/AIDS patients seem to corroborate some of the findings that Jung (1960) observed. Dying has its onset long before actual death and changes of the personality may precede death by quite a long time. Jung says that the unconscious psyche is not so much interested in death as in how one dies and whether or not the attitude of consciousness is adjusted to dying. This conscious attitude toward death, separation and loss is one of the most critical issues in the dying process (Bowlby 1981; Gordon 1993).

Over the years it has become clear what so many HIV/AIDS patients mean when they say 'HIV is the best thing that has ever happened to me'. On the surface it is a crazy statement but when the meaning is explored in psychotherapy one discovers that it is really about the person beginning to live their own life – not the life that they think should be lived or that others think they should live, but the life they were meant to live. The psyche begins to set right what has been wrong. A shift in attitude and consciousness begins to take place. Frequently these individuals begin to make the most of their lives. They consolidate relationships and discard what is no longer needed in their emotional life. They not only go about completing unfinished business, they begin to live from the essence of life and connect with it.

Lives are given new meaning by the fact of death. The psyche wants wholeness. Specifically, patients do more of the things they have wanted, but had not allowed themselves to do. Frequently individuals demonstrate a more open willingness to acknowledge their own human pain and suffering as well as their longings, desires, limitations and choices. As the patient moves closer to their own sense of self, family, friends and lovers are confronted with themselves and their own lives and their own limitations and their own mortality. It would appear that the dying patient elicits in others the threat to their existence and the meaning they ascribe to their own lives. If individuals are to die content, they must each live the task of becoming completely the person they were meant to be (Keys 1981).

How the patient, lovers, family and friends deal with and live the remainder of time before death is often the major issue, particularly because there is only a remainder. As human beings we long for images that are going to help us face as honestly as possible our own lives and in this case, the crises initiated by HIV/AIDS. The psyche needs images and metaphors. They help us see, feel and acknowledge our hopes, our pain, our anger and our grief. Images help us to face and bring into focus that which is unspeakable. Images, stories and words help us to endure and to enter more deeply into our experience (Downing 1989).

During those states of free-floating attention so necessary in psycho-therapy one is often reminded of Monette's *Borrowed Times* (1988) and of Bosnak's *Dreaming with an AIDS Patient* (1989). They both speak so beautifully of the importance of images and of how they help us to live and face HIV/AIDS loss. Monette tells of how, toward the end of his lover's life, they read Plato's *Apology* and *Phaedo* together: 'When you have the time to read a little Plato, when the other half of you wants to do it as much as you do, nobody wastes a moment worrying that he's wasting time' (p 299). 'We read to see how a man of honour faces death without lies' (p 303). Bosnak describes how, at the very end of his patient's life, he visits him in the hospital and reads to him out of his dream book. He gives back to him his own images, reverberating his own creation, his own internal creative life.

Downing (1981, 1991: 12) reminds us that the poets offer us models of living and of facing death that are complex and diverse enough to do justice to individual differences. Like myths, poetry takes us out of our singular vision and shows us the dangers of trying to impose a single model upon the individual that may prevent someone from living their own dying and their death. The poets, she says, remind us that 'death is rarely completing, that many die unreconciled – in fear, anger, denial – that is part of what death is, an intrusion into life that is part of life'.

Life has an end and that end is death; it is dying that is so difficult. There are so many times when, listening to HIV/AIDS patients, one is reminded of Freud (1957) and his 1937 essay 'Analysis Terminable and Interminable'. In that essay, written just before the end of his life, he talks about the last and most difficult task of analysis and in life (especially for men), which is overcoming hatred and fear of the feminine, of dependency, of passivity and of death. This task requires the letting go of control and of the heroic masculine ego. It requires surrendering the body to the ever-increasing illness and physical and emotional dependence upon the health care system and upon one's closest friends. It is dissolution and a surrender to acknowledging the duality that we both hate and long for full union and return to the womb, to return to a good mother and to that fantasized symbiotic feeling when we were safe and when we imagine that our every wish and desire was met and acknowledged (Downing 1989). To be human is to long for such dependency and union and to be in conflict with both Eros and Thanatos.

HIV/AIDS is a crisis of individuation. It requires the person to live their life as if they are going to live forever, yet knowing that they may not even live till the setting sun. Some can respond to the crisis as a challenge and emerge with newly found strengths, positive attitudes and coping skills. Identity can be consolidated as a true sense of self; new depth and love can be found in relationships with family, partners and friends; and new meaning may be derived from the seemingly unjust and senseless.

IMPLICATIONS FOR CLINICAL PRACTICE

Whether the person will die as he/she has lived or whether he/she will accept the challenge of this crisis depends much upon their early childhood experience involving separation (Bowlby 1981; Gordon 1993). In our work with HIV/AIDS patients we must help them examine earlier real or imagined experiences with loss and assist them to discover their own inner unconscious resources in order to make them conscious and accessible to daily life.

One cannot overemphasize the importance of hope. Hope maintains the motivation to make active efforts to enhance health, to comply with medical management, to strengthen the social support system and thus to live longer. Hope and anxiety are emotions that relate us to the future (Solomon & Mead 1987; Kast 1991).

As psychotherapists, if we do not have hope for the patient with HIV/ AIDS or for those who are left behind, that they can come to terms with death and dying and be able to live with the possibility that they may not, then we run the risk as they do of sinking into despair, a despair that brings with it gloom, depression and hopelessness and draws death about itself quickly. We must support the patient's struggle for hope by supporting something vital to the quality of life and to discover meaning.

As psychotherapist and health care professionals we are healers. We become involved in the lives of our patients. We too must find our hope in the hopeless. One of the many challenges in HIV/AIDS work is to remember why we became healers in the first place. This work demands that we go beyond the traditional boundaries of the consulting room. Paradoxically, in this work, we must remember and be aware of, as if we could ever forget, our own pain and loss and our defence mechanisms. We must develop a defensive armour to be able to ward off our own sense of impotence and profound sadness at watching so many young people die and at not being able to master mortality. Without such an awareness of health defence mechanisms our personal and professional lives suffer, as well as our patients.

There are many lessons to be learned from HIV/AIDS. We learn about turning toward the unconscious and trusting the process to heal and to find a creative solution that has been out of conscious awareness. As both patients and healers we learn that the pain of loss never goes away. However, it provides a window to the self and we can only hope to value the living and honour the dying and to love and live our lives more fully in the present.

Lastly, one is reminded of Asclepius, the Greek god of healing. As psychotherapists and physicians he is our god, a god who had also experienced death, a god who learned that human mortality cannot be avoided. Asclepius, so Downing (1989) and Meier (1989) tell us, was the son of Apollo and Coronis. Coronis, after she became pregnant by Apollo, wished to marry and have a father for her son. Apollo was rageful about her unfaithfulness. At about the time that the child was to be delivered, Apollo appeared and in a jealous outburst set Coronis and her bridegroom and friends on fire. Just at that moment, he realized that her son was his son so he cut open Coronis's womb and rescued the child, Asclepius. His birth was a birth in death. Later, Asclepius rescued two mortals from Hades, angering Zeus who slew him with a thunderbolt. He was made a god and immortal, and a shrine was built in Epidaurus. There the sick, the maimed and the ill came to be healed. To be cured they lay upon the stone couch to dream. However, they learned at Epidaurus that to be healed by Asclepius meant that he could give simply the time needed to prepare for a death that would inevitably come, a death that inevitably comes to all of us – ready or not, willing or not.

REFERENCES

Baker B & Wheelwright J (1982) Analysis with the aged. In M Stein (ed) *Jungian Analysis*, London: Open Court pp 256–74

Biller R & Rice S (1990) Experiencing multiple loss of persons with AIDS: grief and bereavement issues *Health Soc Work* **15**: 183–290

Blencher MJ (1993) Psychoanalysis and HIV disease *Contemp Psychoanal* **29**: 61–80

Bosnak R (1989) *Dreaming with an AIDS-patient* Boston: Shambala

Bowlby J (1971) *Attachment and Loss, Vol 1: Attachment* Harmondsworth: Pelican

Bowlby J (1975) *Attachment and Loss, Vol 2: Loss* Harmondsworth: Pelican

Bowlby J (1981) *Attachment and Loss, Vol 3: Loss: Sadness and Depression* Harmondsworth: Pelican

Cohen F & Lazarus RS (1973) Active coping processes, coping dispositions, and recovery from surgery *Psychosom Med* **35**: 375–89

Dane BO (1989) Anticipatory mourning of middle-aged parents of adult children with AIDS *Family Soc* **72**: 108–15

Dilly JW, Pies C & Helquist M (eds) (1989) *Face to Face: a Guide to AIDS Counseling* San Francisco: AIDS Health Project, University of California

Downing C (1981) Your old men shall dream dreams. In J-R Staude (ed) *Wisdom and Age: The Adventure of Later Life* Berkeley, CA: Ross pp 169–86

Downing C (1989) *Myths and Mysteries of Same Sex Love* New York: Continuum

Downing C (1991) A love song: *paper presented at the I Int Congress Biopsychosocial Aspects of HIV Disease* (Amsterdam)

Freud A (1960) A discussion of Dr John Bowlby's paper 'Grief and Mourning in Infancy and Early Childhood' *Psychoanal Study Child* **15**: 53–62

Freud S (1917) Trauer und Melancholie *Int Z Artz Psychoanal* **4**: 288–301

Freud S (1957) Analysis Terminable and Interminable. In E Jones (ed) *Collected Papers Vol 5* London: Hogarth Press pp 316–57

Geis SB, Fuller RL & Rush J (1986) Lovers of AIDS victims: psychosocial stresses and counseling needs *Death Stud* **10**: 43–53

Gordon R (1978) *Dying and Creating: A Search for Meaning* London: Society of Analytical Psychology

Gordon R (1993) *Bridges: Metaphors for Psychic Processes* London: Karnac

Hildebrand HP (1992) A patient dying of AIDS *Int Rev Psychoanal* **19**: 457–69

Jung CG (1956) Symbols of Transformation *Collected Works Vol 5* Princeton: Princeton University Press

Jung CG (1960) Stages of Life *Collected Works Vol 8* Princeton: Princeton University Press pp 387–403

Jung CG (1960) The Soul and Death *Collected Works Vol 8* Princeton: Princeton University Press pp 404–15

Jung CG (1966) Two Essays on Analytical Psychology *Collected Works Vol 7* Princeton: Princeton University Press

Kast V (1991) *Joy, Inspiration and Hope* College Station, Texas: Texas A&M University Press

Keys M (1981) The last years: life and death. In JR Staude (ed) *Wisdom and Age: The Adventure of Later Life* Berkeley, CA: Ross pp 169–86

Klein M (1989) *Poets for Life: Seventy-six Poets Respond to AIDS* New York: Persea

Klein S & Fletcher W (1986) Gay grief: an examination of its uniqueness brought to light by the AIDS crisis *J Psychosoc Oncol* **4**: 15–25

Kubler-Ross E (1969) *On Death and Dying* New York: Macmillan

Liberman MH (1975) Adaptive processes in late life. In N Datan & LH Ginsberg (eds) *Life-span Developmental Psychology: Normative Life Crises* London: Academic Press pp 135–59

Lindemann E (1944) Symptomatology and management of acute grief *Am J Psychiatry* **101**: 141–8

Macks J (1989) The psychological needs of people with AIDS. In JW Dilly, C Pies & M Helquist (eds) *Face to Face: A Guide to AIDS Counselling* San Francisco: AIDS Health Project, University of California pp 2–14

Mansson SA (1992) Dead-end or turning point: on homosexuality and coping with HIV *J Psychol Hum Sexual* **5**: 157–76

May R (1953) *Man's Search for Himself* New York: Signet

May R, Angel E & Ellenberger HF (1958) *Existence* New York: Touchstone

May R (1969) *Existential Psychology* New York: Random House

McCain NL & Gramling LS (1992) Living with dying: Coping with HIV disease *Issues Ment Health Nurs* **13**: 271–83

Meier CA (1989) *Healing, Dream and Ritual* Einsiedeln: Daimon

Meyers WA (1987) Age, rage, and the fear of AIDS *J Geriatr Psychiatry* **20**: 125–40

Monette P (1988) *Borrowed Times* London: Collins Harvill

Moss D (1992) Introductory thoughts: hating in first person plural: the example of homophobia *Am Imago* **49**: 277–91

O'Neil M (1989) Grief and bereavement in AIDS and aging *Generations* **13**: 80–2

Ramos AC (1989) Una enfermedad que irrumpe: el SIDA (Proceso psicoanalitico) [An irruptive disease: AIDS (Psychoanalytic process of a patient)] *Rev Psicoanalisis* **46**: 87–102

Sadowey D (1991) Is there a role for the psychoanalytic psychotherapist with a patient dying of AIDS? *Psychoanal Rev* **78**: 199–207

Saynor JK (1988) Existential and spiritual concerns of people with AIDS *J Palliat Care* **4**: 61–5

Schwartzenberg SS (1992) AIDS-related bereavement among gay men: the inadequacy of current theories of grief *Psychotherapy* **29**: 422–9

Schoen K & Schindelman E (1989) AIDS and bereavement *J Gay Lesbian Psychother* **1**: 117–20

Solomon GF & Mead SCW (1987) Considerations in the treatment of the gay patient with AIDS or ARC *Humane Med* **3**: 10–19

Seligman MEP (1975) *Helplessness* San Francisco: Freeman

Sontag S (1988) *AIDS and its Metaphors* London: Penguin

Taylor SE, Helgeson VS, Reed GM & Skokan LA (1991) Self-generated feelings of control and adjustment to physical illness *J Soc Issues* **47**: 91–109

Tillich P (1955) The eternal now. In H Feifel (ed) *The Meaning of Death* New York: McGraw-Hill

Wilmer HA (1991) Dreams of an analysand dying of AIDS. In HA Wilmer (ed) *Closeness in Personal and Professional Relationships* Boston: Shambala pp 49–59

Wilson P (1988) The impact of cultural changes on the internal experience of the adolescent *J Adolesc* **11**: 271–86

Worden JW (1982) *Grief Counseling and Grief Therapy: A Handbook for the Mental Health Practitioner* New York: Springer

Worden JW (1991) Grieving a loss from AIDS *Hospice J* **7**: 143–50

Yalom ID (1980) *Existential Psychotherapy* New York: Basic Books

Winiarski MG (1991) *AIDS-Related Psychotherapy* New York: Pergamon

Zinkin L (1989) On trying to lead a well balanced life. Paper presented to the Society of Analytical Psychology (25 Jan 1989; cassette recording)

CHAPTER 9

Living Wills

Alison Richardson

City Hospital, Edinburgh, UK

People with AIDS, and in particular gay men with AIDS in the early years of the epidemic, have enabled a wider discussion about the processes and decisions that may precede death. There are potentially and actually many ethical dilemmas that face those who are caring for someone with a diagnosis of HIV infection or AIDS. This is obviously true for many other people in similar situations, caring for those with any illness and particularly true for anyone caring for someone who has been diagnosed with a terminal illness. This chapter illustrates what has happened with and for people with HIV infection, but it applies equally to many others who find themselves in a similar situation.

CASE STUDIES

Case 1: Treatment Refusal
....

A young man presented with pneumocystis pneumonia (PCP) in its early stages. His condition was almost certainly treatable with a good prognosis. He refused all treatment, saying that he did not want to live with HIV any longer. He was not psychiatrically ill and seemed to have thought through his decision. Physicians assured themselves that they had given him all the relevant information about the condition and informed him of the likely course of events if he did or did not take treatment. He died peacefully, without treatment, in a short period of time.
....

In this case, many staff were unhappy about the patient's decision to die, as they saw it, prematurely. Many felt that he was still young and that

Grief and AIDS. Edited by L. Sherr.
©1995 John Wiley & Sons Ltd.

he should continue to fight. The patient felt that he had no quality of life, having lost his job and having no partner, no close family and few friends. Although his physical state was reasonable, he felt that he had no reason to live and did not want to spend some months or years having repeated admissions to hospital and becoming progressively more ill. Assessment might have shown him to be clinically depressed, in which case it might have been right not to accept his decision to refuse treatment, but he appeared to have thought everything through in a rational fashion and therefore his decision was respected. This was hard on staff who had known him for many years as an asymptomatic patient. Their desire that he should live longer and their conviction that he still had something to live for was greater than his own.

Case 2: Decision Making

A young man, who had cytomegalovirus (CMV) and had lost much of his sight, decided that he had had enough and that he wanted all treatment stopped. He had been taking vast quantities of drugs for a considerable time and felt that his whole life was dominated by the virus and by his various treatments. If his CMV treatment was stopped, he would almost certainly have gone blind. After discussion, the patient agreed to continue his CMV treatment, but stopped everything else. At a later date he restarted other treatments, such as PCP prophylaxis, but refused a brain biopsy, which might have shown that he had a treatable condition.

With this patient, his discussion with staff and family resulted in a change of mind about treatment. He was persuaded at least to continue treatment for his CMV retinitis. A change in his mood at a later date resulted in his recommencement of other treatments. This man also made an informed decision not to have an intrusive investigation (brain biopsy) although there was a chance that this would have led to further prolongation of life.

Case 3: Quality of Life

A woman with two children became permanently hospitalized. She was blind and suffering some discomfort. She was repeatedly offered opiates to make her more comfortable. She knew that taking opiates might accelerate her death and consistently refused them. All around her felt that she had no quality of life but her wish not to have opiates was respected.

Case 4: Conflicting Opinions

A young woman was dying with untreatable oesophageal candida. She was unable to swallow and was in considerable pain. In order to keep the pain under control, increasing amounts of opiates were prescribed, to the extent that she was virtually comatose. Her family objected, accusing the physician of killing her. The patient herself was in no state to express her opinion. Reluctantly, the physician reduced her opiates to the point that the patient became more alert, but also in pain. On seeing the result, the family asked for her medication to be increased again. She died peacefully soon after.

Case 5: Coming to Terms with Death

A young drug user presented with *Mycobacterium* infection. He was very ill; this was his third AIDS-defining infection and he had had AIDS for three years. He was interested only in receiving more and more opiate medication and made it clear to the staff that he wanted to spend the rest of his life 'stoned' and preferably asleep. Some staff had great difficulty in accepting his preferred method of coping. They felt that he should be talking about the illness and 'coming to terms' with it. The refusal of more opiates, on the grounds that he was not suffering pain, arguably caused more psychological distress and anger in the patient. He never talked to anyone about how he felt about his impending death.

Learning from Experience

In three of the above cases, the attitudes of staff and others towards the use of pain-killing medication caused problems. The ethical problems surrounding the use of pain-killing medication are even more problematic than the use or non-use of other treatments. Staff attitudes may have a powerful effect on what treatment is regarded as acceptable. In Case 3, all those who cared for the patient were concerned that she had no quality of life and they would have felt happier seeing her in a coma, than seeing her struggling through each day, not able to see and barely able to communicate. Judgements about quality of life in others are perilous. This lady was able to make her own judgement and, though it differed from that of every one else, it had to be respected. She did not herself complain; rather those caring for her, family and staff alike, suffered in watching her and wished for her release.

Pain relief was again problematic in Case 4, partly because the family did not understand what pain the patient would be suffering without opiate medication. The patient herself had not had the opportunity to pronounce on the matter. If she had, it might still have been incumbent on the physician to show why he was prescribing as he did.

In Case 5, attitudes of staff and others towards drug use intruded. There is often a prevailing attitude that it is better for patients to deal with their problems and to come to terms with their illness. For many of those infected through drug use, their response to psychological pain in their lives has been to take drugs. There is little reason for them to change this habitual coping mechanism when they are dying.

Experience has, however, shown that it may be easier for drug users to obtain opiate medication than for others, who may also wish to deal with the psychological distress of this disease by taking drugs. As an example of this, a young woman with AIDS, who had been infected heterosexually by her drug-using partner, was admitted to the ward with a painful infection. She had never used illicit drugs herself. She was put on opiate medication to deal with the pain of her condition. As the infection resolved, staff felt that she was being very resistant to having the medication withdrawn. Lengthy discussion among the multi-disciplinary team elucidated the fact that, had she been a known drug user, there would have been very little concern about this, and much less pressure to withdraw the medication.

These examples show that staff may be more or less likely to acquiesce to requests for opiate medication when the patient is a drug user than when the patient is homosexually, heterosexually or otherwise infected. It need hardly be said that the risk behaviour of those who are infected should have no part in decisions about medical care.

Case 6: 'Do Not Resuscitate' Orders

Some people feel that they want everything possible to be done to keep them alive, and it is only through good clinical discussion that patients may realize that interventions in certain situations may be both futile and undignified.

. . . .

A young woman expressed the desire that her life should be prolonged as long as possible. She had particularly said that she would want both ventilation and cardiopulmonary resuscitation (CPR). She was dying with both respiratory and cardiac failure. CPR would clearly have been futile and was not carried out.

. . . .

This case illustrates the dilemmas surrounding 'Do Not Resuscitate' orders.

Case 7: Family Interventions
. . . .
A young man repeatedly expressed his wish to have a post-mortem investigation after his death, so that he could feel he would be doing something to contribute to further knowledge of the disease. This was documented in his medical notes. His partner, also with AIDS, knew of this wish and agreed with him. After his death his family vetoed this option and the investigation was not carried out.
. . . .

These case histories illustrate a number of important dilemmas for carers, where patients have expressed particular wishes about treatment. Cases 1 to 6 give some indication of the difficulties that physicians and others face when the patient or family express wishes that are contrary to medical opinion. The last case is particularly important in indicating the conflict which may arise between the wishes of families and those of 'significant others', which arises most frequently in the case of gay men and their partners and families. The case studies all indicate how hard it may be for clinical carers to accept the decisions of patients and potentially those close to them. They also convey the importance of assessing the patient's ongoing state of mind when he/she is making decisions about treatment and of sustaining ongoing dialogue with patients about the potential results of these decisions.

Decisions of families or staff on all these matters, when the patient is unable to express their own wishes, are made based on a number of factors: familiarity with the person and his/her wishes, experience with similar medical states, technological expertise and also value judgements. Such value judgements are necessarily made by others, when the patient is no longer able to express their own wishes.

LIVING WILLS

Living wills or 'Advance Directives' allow a person to express their wishes in advance of serious illness. They may be very explicit, for instance, in saying 'If I am diagnosed by my (named) physician as being in a persistent vegetative state, I do not want either intravenous fluids or tube feeding, but I do want everything to be done to keep me comfortable'. Such a directive specifies not only the medical condition and specific interventions but also a specific doctor who is to make the diagnosis. At the other end of the spectrum, a person may leave instructions that everything possible should be done for them, without specifying either condition or treatment. The middle ground lies where less specific scenarios are expressed with options saying that either they do or do not want their lives prolonged as long as possible.

The Terence Higgins Trust in England, in collaboration with the Centre for Medical Law and Ethics, has developed a form which can be used.

Three different scenarios are given as shown below, with the same two different choices in terms of treatment.

Scenario 1: Physical Illness

If I have a physical illness from which there is no likelihood of recovery, and it is so serious that my life is nearing its end. . .

Scenario 2: Permanent Mental Impairment

If my mental functions become permanently impaired with no likelihood of improvement and the impairment is so severe that I do not understand what is happening to me, and I have a physical illness. . .

Scenario 3: Permanent Unconsciousness

If I become permanently unconscious with no likelihood of regaining consciousness. . .

For each of the different scenarios, the same two statements about choice of treatment are given:

A   I wish to be kept alive for as long as reasonably possible using whatever forms of medical treatment are available.
B   I do not wish to be kept alive by medical treatment. I wish medical treatment to be limited to keeping me comfortable and free from pain.

A further section allows the person to specify any wishes that he/she might have with regard to particular medical treatments. This section might be used, for instance, specifically to exclude or include such treatments as tube feeding or ventilation.

Section 3 provides the ability to override the earlier stated choices temporarily, so that a named person can be with the patient before death.

Finally there is a section in which the patient can appoint a proxy to participate in decisions about medical care on the patient's behalf if he/she is unable to do so.

In AIDS, this last section may be particularly important, since, as in Case 7 above, the person closest to the dying patient may not be a member of the family, but the family may still feel that they have a greater right to make such decisions than, for instance, a gay partner. This is not only true for gay men, however. In other cases, patients have specifically excluded their blood or marital next of kin from making decisions for them and have named people other than husbands, wives, mothers, fathers, etc. as their next of kin.

People with HIV infection and with AIDS are obviously not alone in their concern with what will happen to them when they are dying, as a number of research projects in the USA have shown. It is probably true to say that people with AIDS have brought many of the issues to the fore in the past ten years and have informed the debate about the ethics of continuing or discontinuing treatment for those who are terminally ill. Most people, if asked, seem to have a view on whether or not they would wish a number of treatments, given different states of illness.

RESEARCH FINDINGS

In the USA decisions to withhold or to withdraw treatment seem still to be more often discussed than in the UK (Jennett 1987). The Patient Self Determination Act in the USA (Omnibus Reconciliation Act (1990)) requires that all hospitals have a policy on living wills and that all admitted patients should be asked if they have one. Most states have legislated for living wills and/or durable states of attorney (where a proxy decision maker is appointed to make decisions about health care, if the patient himself/herself is incompetent to do so). Some states exclude particular treatments such as intravenous fluids and tube feeding. It has been suggested by the American College of Physicians (1992) that such exclusions might be overturned by the courts in the USA as a violation of the patient's rights. In both the USA and Europe, such treatments are those which have caused most public concern, with cases such as that of Tony Bland in the UK being taken through the courts to establish the right of physicians to withdraw feeding. Tony Bland had been crushed in the Hillsborough disaster and was in a persistent vegetative state for four years. His parents and doctors were finally permitted to withdraw feeding after his case was taken to the House of Lords.

In contrast with the USA, the UK has no legislation pertaining to living wills. The *Bulletin of Medical Ethics* (1993), reporting on the House of Lords debate about Tony Bland, suggested that the common law might find living wills to be valid, even in the absence of statute. Two of the Lords (Lord Keith of Kinkel and Lord Goff of Chieveley) made the following points:

1 It is unlawful to administer treatment to an adult who is conscious and of sound mind without his consent.

2 This extends to the situation where the person, anticipating a condition where he might be unable to give consent, has given clear instructions that in such an event 'he is not to be given medical care, including *artificial feeding*' [author's emphasis].
3 Where (2) applies, special care may be necessary to ensure that the prior refusal of consent is still applicable.

A number of important studies have been carried out in the USA into preferences for treatment in the general population and patients, as well as in people with AIDS. Reviewing these and other relevant literature, a number of crucial components emerge.

Choices about Illness and Treatment

Does the person have specific views about any of the following?

1 The prolongation of treatment in general.
2 Specific treatments, e.g. tube feeding, chemotherapy, ventilation, pain control.
3 Particular disorders, e.g. disfiguring complaints, those that might cause blindness, illnesses that may or may not cause death slowly or quickly, those that cause cognitive impairment.
4 Resuscitation, in the event of cardiac or respiratory failure.
5 Intrusive or potentially painful investigations.
6 Post-mortem investigations.

Choices about Control

Who should make the decision about any of the above if the patient cannot? There seems to be a consensus that the patient's wishes, expressed when cognitively unimpaired, should be overriding. *The American College of Physicians Ethics Manual* (1992) suggests that decisions should be made on the basis of advance directives, substituted judgements (proxy decision makers) and the best interests of the patient, *in that order of priority*.

Such judgements are helpful, but do not address the reality of the fact that most people neither make living wills, nor provide legally binding advance directives which appoint a proxy decision maker. They also may ignore the fact, particularly in illnesses such as AIDS, that advancing medical technology may make previously expressed wishes redundant.

A number of studies in the USA have attempted to examine the views of a number of populations with regard to living wills. One of these early studies was carried out in 1986 with 118 young homosexual men with an AIDS diagnosis (Steinbrook et al 1986).

This study was important in beginning to look at the wishes of patients should they develop different conditions and asked very specific questions concerned with (a) awareness of life-sustaining treatments; (b) preferences with regard to specific treatments in one condition: pneumocystis pneumonia (PCP), complicated or not by cognitive impairment; (c) preferences with regard to discussions with doctors about life-sustaining treatment; (d) their wishes with regard to others making decisions for them if they were unable to do so themselves; (e) actions already taken to put any of the above into operation; (f) estimates of survival in specific situations. The study also attempted to look at the consistency of patients' choices over time. A large number of demographic details were also collected.

In this particular study, people who had already experienced PCP were more likely to have discussed life-sustaining treatment with their doctor, than people who had not. Nearly three-quarters of the patients said that they would like to discuss these matters with their doctor, but only one-third had done so. It was unclear from the study why the others had not. Interestingly, patients who reported a negative emotional reaction to discussing life-sustaining treatments were as likely as others to want such discussions. It is almost certainly the case that clinical carers often refrain from raising these subjects out of concern that such discussion will cause distress to the patient.

With regard to the treatment of PCP, 95% of the patients expressed the wish that they would want to be hospitalized and given antibiotics, 55% wanted intensive treatment with mechanical ventilation and 46% wanted cardiopulmonary resuscitation, but the patients generally overestimated the likelihood of survival in specific situations. Their mean estimate was of 56% survival when the patient required intubation, while the authors reported an actual survival rate at that time of 14% (Murray et al 1984).

The patients had distinct views about who should initiate such discussions (patient or physician) and about when they should occur (as out-patients, in-patients or when AIDS was diagnosed). The majority wanted such discussions as out-patients, once they had got to know their physician. Common sense suggests that this is probably the right time for such discussions to take place and easier for both physician and patient. Most people would want to discuss such painful topics with someone that they knew and trusted rather than with a stranger. Waiting to discuss it until ill, hospitalized or nearer death is more likely to cause distress to both carer and patient.

In this group of homosexual men, 47% wanted their partners or friends to act as proxy if they became mentally incompetent, 32% wanted family members and 14% their physicians. A total of 67% had provided advance directives of some kind or another, 49% through having at least discussed it with families, but fewer (38%) had made a living will and fewer still (28%) had executed a durable power of attorney for health care.

A more recent study of HIV-positive individuals (Teno et al 1990) indicated that 68% of the 1031 patients studied knew about advance directives, but only 28% had acted upon the knowledge.

Another study, conducted in 1991 with out-patients and with members of the general public in Boston showed a similarly high awareness of the purpose of living wills. It seems unlikely that such awareness would have been found if the same study had been undertaken in 1986 among these populations. A large majority expressed their desire to have discussion with their doctors about treatments if they were in a number of different terminal states (Emanuel et al 1991). About 90% of all those interviewed (405 out-patients and 102 members of the general public) said that they would wish to make advance directives, but less than 20% had done so. As many as 59% said that they would like to discuss the matter with their physician, but in fact only 5% had done so. Similarly, 78% wished to appoint a proxy decision maker, but only 8% had designated one in writing and, although 57% wanted a document specifying future care, only 7% had one.

The study presented a number of different scenarios and a number of different interventions. The out-patients refused life-sustaining treatments in 71% of their choices: coma with a chance of recovery (57%), persistent vegetative state (85%), dementia (79%) and dementia with a terminal illness (87%). Averaged over these scenarios the rate of refusal for specific interventions was major surgery (76%), dialysis and artificial nutrition (74%), mechanical respiration, cardiopulmonary resuscitation and blood transfusion (73%), intravenous fluids (71%).

It is almost impossible to compare the responses of the AIDS patients in 1985 with the responses of these out-patients and members of the general public who were less ill and certainly not terminally so. It does seem that the AIDS patients overall were more likely to wish to have interventions. This might simply be because the situation was not hypothetical for the AIDS patients; they were already sick and likely to die within a relatively short period when asked about their preferences for treatment. The ambivalence that people experience in this situation is frequently illustrated in day-to-day work with people who are HIV-infected. When a patient is well, has never been hospitalized and has not observed the effect of the progression of the disease on other people, he/she may make very different decisions than those made after repeated admissions for infections and invasive treatments and after watching contemporaries die. This distinction is important in ongoing work with HIV-infected people because they may change their minds about what kind of interventions they want in different situations, or indeed who they would want to make decisions for them if they became mentally incompetent themselves. In the Steinbrook study 9% of the patients had changed their mind at some point about life-sustaining treatment and 22% had changed their mind about who should be their proxy decision maker.

It might be hypothesized that younger people with longer life expectancy are more likely to want interventions. Equally it might be that those who are young and in good health might find it easier to refuse, having had less experience and knowledge about what happens in terminal illness. In some scenarios in the Boston study, there were some indications that young patients were more likely to refuse interventions such as mechanical respirations when in a persistent vegetative state than were older people. State of health had some bearing on the attitudes of the patients with, for instance, 71% of those in good health refusing antibiotics if they had dementia compared with 59% of those in poor health. This was not found in the study of AIDS patients, where there was no association between state of health and preference for mechanical ventilation.

Neither study showed association between wish for intervention and any other demographic variables, including state of health. It can only be concluded that there are no reliable predictors, at the current time, of what an individual's wish for medical intervention will be under different circumstances and at different times. Living wills and advance directives therefore seem to be a way for people to do as much as they can to ensure that their wishes are respected, even if they become unable to express them themselves. It also seems clear that the majority of people have a view about what they would like to happen under different circumstances of illness, although it is possible that those views change over time, depending on circumstances. Legislation in the USA has obviously raised awareness about this topic and there seems little doubt that, if asked, the vast majority of people believe that making advance directives is desirable. So, if most people want to make a living will, what stops them?

In the Boston study, one of the most frequently cited reasons for failing to have an advance directive was the expectation that the physician should take the initiative in raising the subject. One of the least reported barriers was the sensitivity of the subject for the patient. Steinbrook and colleagues (1986) also made the point that their results refuted such objections to discussing life-sustaining treatments as the sensitivity of the subject and that patients do not want such discussions.

Psychological Mechanisms

It seems reasonable to suggest that the same psychological mechanism is in operation that often prevents people from making wills which dispose of their property. It seems not unreasonable (though simplistic, in psychological terms) to hypothesize that denial of the possibility of death plays a part. It often seems that patients can grasp intellectually the fact that they are dying, but that emotionally it continues to seem unreal. One recent example of this was a patient who had already made a will before being diagnosed with HIV infection. He was physically well at that time but became profoundly depressed and tried to commit suicide. Three years later, after it was clear that he was becoming ill, he expressed a desire to change this will. Although he frequently talked about it, he never did anything about it, saying that there was plenty of time to do so. Another contribution to his failure to redraft his will was the considerable reluctance of family, friends, physicians and psychologist to confront him with the reality of his own imminent death, given his catastrophic reaction to the news that he was infected with HIV.

TALKING TO THE PATIENT

It is clear that ongoing dialogue with the patient about treatments and prognosis is essential for the patient to make informed choices about treatment. Advances in the medical management of some conditions may affect decisions about what treatments to accept. When the 1985 study was carried out, there were no treatments for some AIDS-related conditions which are now eminently treatable. For instance, reliable diagnosis and reliable and effective treatment of dementia associated with HIV infection might radically change patients' attitudes to life-sustaining treatment. This is the condition, in the author's experience, about which most people express fear.

Dialogue about the process of dying and death may become both easier and more difficult for clinical carers as they get to know patients; easier because they get to know through experience what kind of attitudes, problems and fears the patients have, more difficult because carers may come to know their patients much more intimately than in other disease processes. It is not uncommon for physicians and others in the clinical professions to look after their patients for many years; the carers are often of the same age as those they are treating or may identify with them in other ways so that it is sometimes difficult to retain professional detachment and to accept the patient's negative attitude towards treatment when their own belief is that treatment will help them in some way.

Often carers, whether friends, families or clinical carers, feel that they know what the person would have wanted and discussions take place around the 'quality of life' of the person, who may be comatose or unable to express their wishes through cognitive impairment. Substitute decision making, however, does not necessarily accurately reflect the wishes of patients with regard to resuscitation. In a study of this, there was as little as 59% agreement, in some scenarios, between the patient's expressed wishes and those that a proxy would have given (Seckler et al 1991). Appointed proxies should both always know that they have been appointed as proxy and know what the patient himself/herself would want in different situations. Proxy judgements should obviously be made on the basis of knowledge about the patient's wishes and not on the decisions that the proxies would make for themselves, if they found themselves in a similar situation.

IMPLICATIONS FOR PRACTICE

First of all, carers should probably appreciate that most of us will have views about treatment options when we are in different states of illness. In the Boston study, the majority seemed to prefer the topic to be raised by their physician. It is also evident that fewer people make arrangements than would like to do so. The institutionalized nature of hospital care often makes people feel that they are not in control and patients may become reactive to the clinical carers, rather than continuing to take an active role. It is probably often easier for the patient to discuss these issues with clinical carers than with family, friends, lovers, etc., since patients may perceive that their clinical carers are less emotionally involved.

Clinical carers have a crucial role to play in raising these subjects with their patients, preferably at a stage in illness when it can be regarded by both parties as hypothetical, rather than as an immediate problem. It should not be assumed that those who are predicted to have a negative emotional reaction to such discussions do not want to participate in them.

Some decisions about treatment are obviously easier to make than others. There are fewer problems associated with the administration of antibiotics than there are with pain relief, for instance. Staff attitudes are often important in determining treatment and this can only be dealt with through discussion. Moral and religious beliefs of staff may affect the kind of treatment that a patient receives and it is important for carers to discuss these with a patient, so that the patient has the choice of transferring their care to another.

It is important that carers continue to be aware of the possibility of changing moods and minds. It is not enough to bring up these topics on one occasion and assume that the person's wish today will be the same in a week or a month or a year. Having discussed the matter once, it becomes easier to keep checking that the person's wish remains the same. Advance Directive Forms, such as those produced by the Terence Higgins

Trust, make the subject easier to raise, but should not be used as a bureaucratic substitute for ongoing discussion with the patient.

GRIEVING

HIV-positive individuals, like any others suffering from a terminal illness, differ in their ability to cope with the probability of their own deaths. Some choose to deny that possibility entirely, others are able to confront it, but more often, perhaps, they move between one and the other at different times. Most face the possibility or probability of death at some time during their illness and grieve for their own lost lives and for those whom they know they will be leaving behind. Many of those suffering from this disease have had many years to think about the where, when and how of their own death. Discussion of these may be painful, but for many people and for their relatives, it seems to bring a sense of relief. Terminally ill people and their loved ones may enter into a conspiracy of silence and unrealistic hope which raises barriers in communication. For the dying patient, and people who care about them, whether death is days or months away, decision making about disposition of assets, about how the person wants to die, about treatments in different eventualities is almost always painful and upsetting. However, for many people, it is a relief to be able to acknowledge impending death. Patients and those close to them can confront the possibilities and realities of the situation with sadness and grief but in the knowledge that they still have some control over what happens to them. Living wills are one way in which this important developmental step can be taken.

REFERENCES

American College of Physicians (1992) Position Paper: American College of Physicians Ethics Manual: Third Edition *Ann Intern Med* **117**(11): 947–60

Bulletin of Medical Ethics (1993) New advice on resuscitation. March: 5–6

Emanuel LL, Barry MJ, Stoeckle JD et al (1991) Special articles: advance directives for medical care – a case for greater use *N Engl J Med* **324**: 889–95

Jennett B (1987) Decisions to limit treatment *Lancet* **ii**: 787–9

Murray JF, Felton CP, Garay SM et al (1984) Pulmonary complications of the acquired immunodeficiency syndrome: report of a National Heart, Lung and Blood Institute workshop *N Engl J Med* **310**: 1682–8

Omnibus Reconciliation Act (1990) Title IV, Section 4206 *Congressional Record* October 26: 12 638

Seckler AB, Meier DE, Mulvihill M & Paris BE (1991) Substituted judgement: how accurate are proxy predictions? *Ann Intern Med* **115**: 92–8

Steinbrook R, Lo B, Tirpack J et al (1986) Special report: preferences of homosexual men with AIDS for life sustaining treatment *N Engl J Med* **314**: 457–60

Teno J, Fleishman J, Brock DW & Mor V (1990) The use of formal prior directives among patients with HIV-related diseases *J Gen Intern Med* **5**: 490–4

CHAPTER 10

The Death of a Parent

Frans M. van den Boom

Blood Transfusion Council of the Netherlands Red Cross, The Netherlands

The death of a parent is not something a dependent child expects to experience, yet it is not uncommon. In the Western world approximately 4–5% of children experience the death of a parent before the age of 15 (e.g. Weller et al 1991; Silverman et al 1992). However, there has been relatively little systematic research on children's reactions to parental death and the relation of bereavement in childhood to subsequent psychopathology. This is true for bereavement in childhood in general, as well as for bereavement in children whose parent(s) have died as a result of AIDS. In their bibliography on AIDS-related bereavement and grief, Bergeron and Handley (1992) mention only one case study, by Demb (1989). Since then, a little more information has become available.

In the Western world the AIDS epidemic has not yet dramatically changed the overall epidemiological prevalence of children experiencing the death of a parent. However, in some areas and subpopulations death due to AIDS has become one or even the most important cause of death.

The relationship between AIDS and the impact of parental death might be rather different from that when parental death is due to other factors. First of all, it is not uncommon that both parents and siblings are infected. This fact alone places a heavy burden on the bearing-power of parents, since they are confronted with grief because they are infected themselves, bereft due to the loss of a partner and/or one of the children, and guilt since most childhood HIV is acquired perinatally. Second, for disadvantaged families, HIV adds to an already burdensome litany of issues, such as poverty, racial discrimination, divorce, crime and drug dependence (e.g. Samperi and Ahto 1991; Giaquinto et al 1992; Lipson 1993). Third, the social stigma that still surrounds AIDS and the fact that HIV/AIDS is still associated with socially taboo behaviors, can make disclosure more difficult. Last but not least, in many cases both parents

Grief and AIDS. Edited by L. Sherr.
©1995 John Wiley & Sons Ltd.

are HIV-infected and ultimately die because of AIDS; this creates the much discussed problem of the so-called AIDS orphans.

In the following pages an overview of the literature on childhood bereavement is presented. The following thematic areas are addressed: (a) children's conceptions of death; (b) short- and long-term impact of parental death; (c) form and contents of intervention programs; and (d) determinants of psychological problems. Specific issues concerning parental death due to HIV/AIDS are then addressed.

CHILDREN'S CONCEPTIONS OF DEATH

For adults it is obvious that death is universal (death comes to all), irreversible (death is final) and inevitable (death is due to cessation of internal body functions). Children's conceptions of death are highly dependent on their cognitive development, however. In order to work effectively with children experiencing the death of a parent, it is vital to understand the child's concept of death. Although there is evidence that many children gain mature conceptions of death at an age younger than that predicted by Piaget's model (Prichard and Epting 1991–1992), children's conceptions of death closely parallel Piaget's (1952) successive levels of cognitive development (Moody and Moody 1991).

During the sensorimotor period (birth to 2 years) the concept of death is non-existent or incomplete (Kane 1979; cited in Moody and Moody 1991). During Piaget's preoperational period (years 2 to 6), a child's cognitions are dominated by magical thinking and egocentrism. Consequently, children in this stage magically believe that death can either be avoided or reversed. They conceive of death as reversible and attributable to neither cessation of body functions nor inevitable causes. In this period the young child may become preoccupied with fears centered on the bodily functions of the deceased, such as how the parent can breathe or eat underground. Because the preoperational period is also dominated by egocentrism, the child may ascribe the parent's death to his or her own behavior; thus the child may also feel responsible for causing the death of the parent and consequently feel shame and guilt. In this period it is essential to reassure children that they are not responsible, discuss the reality of death, and repeat the accurate concepts of death.

Through the period of concrete operations (6 or 7 years to 11 or 12 years), children begin to understand the reality of death but do not realize that death is universal and that those around them, including their loved ones, will die some day. Overall, children in this second stage tend to conceptualize death in concrete terms and view death as distant from themselves. Gradually, from the age of 9 or 10, children acquire a more mature understanding of death. Eventually they realize that death is irreversible in nature and that they themselves will ultimately experience it. During this period, sound and honest information is essential. The most vital information is that the dead person will never return.

Formal operational thinking has been related to the development of complex systems of religious and philosophical thought concerning the nature of death and life after death.

THE IMPACT OF PARENTAL DEATH

Those who work with bereaved children must become acquainted not only with how children understand death but also with how they respond to death, so that problem areas can be assessed and alleviated. It is believed that the death of a parent is a uniquely stressful life event that compromises children's short-term and long-term psychosocial development (Rutter 1975; Christ et al 1991; Mireault and Bond 1992; Saler and Skolnick 1992).

Short-Term Impact

The first reaction following the death has been called the 'emotional outcry phase' (Horowitz 1986) or the 'impact phase' (Tyhurst 1957). It is considered to be a phase in which emotional outbreaks occur, often going along with feelings of anxiety and disbelief. A study by Silverman and Worden (1992) showed that 'few children expressed any immediate anger (7%) or relief (4%) when there had been a prolonged illness with considerable suffering. Most children (44%) talked of feeling sad or confused on hearing the news, even when the death was expected. . . . At some point during the day, the majority of children (91%) broke down in tears'.

The children's inner feelings after the death and their associated behavior included crying, insomnia, learning difficulties, and early health problems that reflected the somatization of feelings. Four months after the death, 62% of the children were no longer crying at frequent intervals or with any regularity, which does not mean that the children were detached. Silverman and colleagues (1992) found that during the year following a parent's death, children develop an inner construction of the dead parent by which they maintain the attachment to him or her. This inner representation or construction leads the child to remain in a relationship with the deceased, and this relationship changes as the child matures and as the intensity of the grief lessens. While the loss is permanent

Table 10.1 Depressive symptoms in 38 bereaved children as reported by the children and by their parents (after Weller et al 1991; reproduced by permission)

	Child report (%)	Parent and child report (%)
Dysphoria	53	61
Loss of interest	34	45
Appetite disturbance	21	24
Sleep disturbance	29	32
Psychomotor agitation or retardation	32	37
Fatigue	8	11
Guilt/worthlessness	21	37
Trouble thinking	5	13
Morbid/suicidal ideation	47	61
Diagnosis of major depressive episode	26	37

and unchanging, the process is not. Bereavement should be understood as a cognitive, as well as an emotional, process that takes place in a social context of which the deceased is a part. Working through the loss is not a matter of a breakthrough, but is better described as a dribble of small steps.

Weller and colleagues (1991) evaluated a group of 38 recently bereaved children aged 5 to 12 years, using structured interviews and rating scales. Children and parents were independently and simultaneously evaluated. When the reports of children and parents were combined, one-third (37%) of the children met the DSM–III–R criteria for a major depressive episode. Dysphoria, loss of interest, appetite disturbance, sleep disturbance, psychomotor agitation or retardation, guilt/worthlessness, and morbid/suicidal ideation were each reported by or for at least one-quarter of the bereaved children (Table 10.1).

Long-Term Impact

The effect of early loss has been thought so critical to development, that much research has been devoted to link this experience with adult psychopathology, especially depression. Beginning with Freud, many theorists have suggested that childhood loss may predispose an individual to depression in adulthood. This is understandable since in adult clinical samples, particularly among the depressed, there is an over-representation of the early bereaved. Many clinicians and theorists therefore perceive the loss experience to be a major risk factor for later maladjustment (Mireault and Bond 1992).

However, the available literature is inconclusive with respect to early loss experience and presence of psychological problems in adulthood. The literature is, however, clear in the finding that there is more than one factor at play. Mireault and Bond (1992) report that the bereft group did not differ from the non-bereft group in anxiety and depression. However, the bereaved subjects scored higher than did controls on their total scores on the perceived vulnerability measure.[1] They suggest that perceived vulnerability may act as a cognitive mediator in the development of depression and anxiety, and conclude that the relationship between parental death in childhood and adult adjustment is complex.

In accordance with this is the finding of Saler and Skolnick (1992) that parental death itself may be an unstable predictor of depression because specific aspects of familial environment and loss situation, in particular the relationship with the surviving parent, may mediate between parental death and depression. Tennant (1988; quoted in Saler and Skolnick 1992), after a review of relevant studies, came to a similar conclusion: while studies of parental death alone showed no significant relationship to later depression, parental problems after any childhood loss would be the most important mediator.

Saler and Skolnick's most important conclusions are:

1 Individuals who reported less opportunity for participation in various activities that are believed to foster the mourning process had higher rates of greater depression or guilty self-reproach.
2 Having a surviving parent characterized by emotional coldness or indifference, correlates among others with higher self-criticism scales.
3 Children of surviving parents described as 'neglectful' or 'affectionate constraint', or 'affectionless control' were more likely than those in the 'optimally-bounded' group to describe depressive experiences of self-criticism.
4 Subjects who experienced maternal death had a poorer sense of well-being and self-confidence than did subjects experiencing paternal death.

Determinants of Psychopathology

Findings such as those by Saler and Skolnick (1992) and Mireault and Bond (1992) highlight the primary importance of environmental and familial factors, including support from and open communication with the surviving parent around issues related to the death. Mental illness following a death seems not so much a consequence of bereavement as of how the bereavement is handled and what happens in the family afterwards. To put it differently: the death of a loved one invariably leads

Table 10.2 Depressive symptoms as a function of the sex of the living parent, the age, sibling position and sex of the child, pre-existing psychiatric disorder, family history of depression, and socioeconomic status (SES)

Sex of the living parent	+ (mother surviving: more depressive symptoms)
Sex of the child	−
Age of the child	−
Sibling position	−
Pre-existing psychiatric disorder in the child	+
Family history of depression	+
Socioeconomic status	+ (higher SES: more depressive symptoms)

to psychological and social stress, but not necessarily to psychiatric symptoms. The ability to deal with this change seems to be the result of the interaction among the social context, the family system and the personal characteristics of those involved.

Weller and colleagues (1991) looked at whether the total number of depressive symptoms varied as a function of the sex of the living parent, the sex of the child, the age of the child, sibling position in the family, pre-existing psychiatric disorder in the child, family history of depression, and socioeconomic status. The results are summarized in Table 10.2.

In their review of the literature Siegel and colleagues (1990) maintained that a child's adjustment to loss is influenced by the extent to which the surviving parent is able to sustain competence in providing support and care for the children, to provide an environment in which the child feels able to express distressing or conflicting thoughts, feelings, and fantasies about the loss, and maintain stability and consistency in the child's environment. The way the surviving parent responds to the child, the availability of social support and subsequent life circumstances make a difference in whether a child develops problems. Rutter (1987) argues that longer-term outcomes are probably less the result of the active stress of the death than of the cumulative stress from the multiple changes that it brings about.

FORM AND CONTENTS OF INTERVENTION PROGRAMS

The importance attached to a stable environment has profound implications for prevention and intervention programs. Considering the above, it is not surprising that so much emphasis is placed upon the role of the remaining parent or a significant other in fostering the children's necessary grief work and resolution of the loss.

Although many will intuitively support these notions, it is important to realize that it is extremely difficult to live up to these requirements. The death of a partner is generally regarded as one of the most stressful life events an adult can experience. The remaining parent not only has to deal with his or her own grief, but has to continue to function as a supporting parent. In a period where maximum efficacy, strength, and availability are needed, many parents find themselves in a time of helplessness and lowered self-esteem due to the loss. Consequently, they have difficulty meeting their children's needs. Thereby one has to realize that working through the loss is a longer-term process of accommodation and adaptation both for children and the remaining parent, which ultimately might result in a satisfying memorialization of the deceased. This requires a double and longer-term effort on the part of the remaining parent. Unfortunately, in the chaos and altered life circumstances that often accompany terminal illness, the surviving spouse may feel it necessary to make changes in family life. Such changes can deprive children of important social support systems that could potentially buffer the impact of loss (e.g. Siegel et al 1990).

The other and brighter side of the coin is that feeling able to meet the children's needs and to be a good parent at this difficult time can greatly enhance the surviving parent's sense of self-esteem and capacity to help their children. Preferably, prevention and intervention programs should support parents as well as children.

In treatment, three important intervention strategies can be distinguished: parent-guidance models, support groups for children, and system/family therapy. Parent-guidance models 'borrow' from family therapy and system therapy but cannot be equated with them. Most of the parent-guidance models are limited in time and do not pretend to address, let alone solve, pre-existing intrapsychic and interpersonal conflicts within the family system. In this context, the distinction that Christ and colleagues (1991) make is relevant. They distinguish between high-risk families, vulnerable families and resilient families. Families in the last category (a) ask for professional help the most easily and (b) are therefore relatively easy to meet psychologically.

This creates the paradoxical situation that 'The individuals with the greatest capacity for self-help often show the least reluctance to call for help from others. Their security in regard to their own autonomous strength frees them to ask for help and to profit from help without feeling that this a sign of weakness. If external support is not available, they are very willing to struggle on their own, but if it is available they use it' (Caplan 1990). This observation was supported in a study by Van den Boom and co-workers (1991), who found that the patients who were coping best sought significantly more professional psychosocial help than those who were coping poorly.

Parent Guidance

In parent-guidance intervention, the primacy remains with the remaining parent. The child's remaining parent will, in most cases, be the most consistently available figure to the child as he or she confronts the many adaptations that, over time, the loss will necessitate (Christ et al 1991). In a sense the surviving parent has to be equipped with information, knowledge and tools to support his or her children. The idea is that the adult helper can guide the parent to understand his or her grief and encourage expression, while at the same time enhancing the ability of these parents to meet their children's heightened needs (Christ et al 1991). This requires parents to be aware that children mourn in a different way than they do, and that the way grief is expressed depends on the developmental stage of the child; moreover, they should know the most common reactions to loss in children and know what to do and say and what to avoid. For example, many parents think that it is better not to discuss the death of the parent; they believe that by doing this, they are protecting their children from the pain and the effects of the death (Siegel et al 1990). They do not realize that, by not addressing the death, they miss the opportunity to correct present anxieties, beliefs and distorted fantasies. As Zambelli and DeRosa (1992) note, it is extremely important to investigate the children's beliefs about death, since they can be extremely troubling and horrifying. Encouraging the children to differentiate between facts and beliefs about death seems to help children gain more control over their fears. The extent to which children can successfully resolve their feelings and grieve appropriately largely depends on correction of their distorted fantasies, and this can best be achieved through open parent–child communication.

Christ and co-workers (1991), Siegel and colleagues (1990) and Melvin and Sherr (1993) point out that when parental death is due to a protracted illness such as AIDS, professionals are presented with the opportunity to attempt primary prevention before children's adjustment problems, or the conditions that lead to such problems, emerge. By intervening before the loss, professionals might avert many problems that arise when the child is inadequately prepared for the death and for the changes in the family environment that immediately follow it. Emphasis is placed on encouraging open communication about the illness and its prognosis, and on maintaining as much stability and predictability in the children's environment as possible.

Child Support Groups

Child support models are not meant to replace but to complement parental support. Their role increases to the extent to which the remaining parent is unable to provide support. When the need of the surviving parent for support in resolving their loss goes unmet, they are less likely to perceive their children's needs and to provide the necessary support for their mourning; the significance of the group will increase accordingly. However, a professional helper or a mutual help group can never replace a supportive parent or the family, since: 'While individual family members have their internalization, or inner representation of the deceased, the family as a whole may also have communal or shared representations' (Silverman et al 1992). Sharing such experiences can be a powerful facilitator in the grief process.

However, the opposite holds true as well; if a family cannot deal with the loss, either the loss is not discussed or the risk impact is followed by negative chain events. 'Parenting functions, which include stimulus buffering, mediation of tension states, modulation of mood and affect states, and empathic perceptions of when and what the child needs to integrate about the death, may become inconsistent and unreliable' (Altschul 1988, cited by Zambelli and DeRosa 1992).

Support groups provide recognition, identification and differentiation. Identification is needed because the support groups are homogeneous in the sense that all the children are bereaved, heterogeneous in the sense that the children carry with them different backgrounds, different coping styles, and different conceptions about death. In a child bereavement group, the availability of the group leader and other children gives the children the opportunity to see and identify with attitudes to death that may be at variance with their own or with those of the surviving parent. 'Since the children receive the stimulus buffering and empathic responses necessary for containing the anxiety associated with their grief responses, this may help to reduce a course of negative chain events' (Zambelli and DeRosa 1992). Additionally, support groups have the potential to bolster self-esteem that is temporarily lowered because of the death, offer an opportunity for education so that children improve their knowledge and cognitive understanding of the death and help bring further meaning to death.

It speaks for itself that it is essential to facilitate a safe place for children to express their feelings unconditionally. Yet, children are often afraid and even unable to recognize and then express their feelings verbally. An effective vehicle to breach the verbal communication barrier and guide the child to his or her natural feelings, is formed by using group techniques such as music therapy, bibliotherapy, art work, game play, role play, body movement in addition to discussion (e.g. Siegel et al 1990; Christ et al 1991; Moody and Moody 1991; Zambelli and DeRosa 1992).

THE FAMILY AND AIDS: INFECTED, UNINFECTED AND AFFECTED

Parental death from other causes than AIDS is primarily dealt with in the nuclear family. In working through the experienced loss, a crucial role is ascribed to the remaining parent, who should provide:

1   Physical and emotional support.
2   An environment in which the child feels able to express distressing or conflicting thoughts, feelings and fantasies about the loss.
3   Stability and consistency in the child's environment.

Basically this presupposes that the familial environment before the death was already characterized by a minimum of structure, openness and consistency.

In the case of AIDS, the majority of children who have one or both parents infected with HIV live or lived in broken/disturbed families. Nicholas and Abrams (1992) address the fact that many HIV-infected children are effectively orphaned prior to the parents' death. 'This phenomenon is best reflected by the living arrangements of HIV-positive children (which we believe parallel those of uninfected siblings): only 45% of all HIV-positive children who received health care in New York during 1990 lived with their biologic parent; 16% lived with a relative; and 33% lived with unrelated foster or adoptive parents. In 1989, 39% of the HIV-positive children born at Harlem hospital went into foster care directly from the newborn nursery because of an inability by the mother to provide adequate care'. Similar findings are reported by Giaquinto and co-workers (1992) and Ronald et al (1993). It comes down to the fact that many of these children live in 'That complex place called poverty, and have a whole range of unmet social, educational and health needs' (Nicholas and Abrams 1992). The implication is that the minimum conditions to provide support to children after the loss of a parent often are absent, at least within the biologic family. 'The combination of a chronic, ultimately lethal disease with serious economic hardship and family and social disintegration has made the daily care of these patients (i.e. women and children with HIV infection) almost impossible' (Heagarty and Abrams 1992).

Moreover, considering the fact that many of the families concerned have a family history of psychiatric disorder and that such a history is one of the determinants of complicated grief, it should not be any surprise that the death of a parent due to AIDS negatively impacts the development of the child, as well as the way in which he or she is supported in the working-through process following the death. Coping abilities are put under even more pressure, if the remaining parent and other siblings are

HIV-infected. Special attention to the problems of young carers, a role to which many of these children are implicitly and slowly condemned, is necessary.

Michaels and Levine (1992) have estimated that in the US by 1992, 18 500 children and adolescents had already been orphaned. By 1996 this number will increase to 45 600 and by the year 2000 to 82 000 orphans. Ankrah (1993) estimates that between 3.1 and 5.5 million children will be orphaned in 10 Eastern and Central African countries alone. 'Neglected in terms of the disruption of relationships with the most significant others, or as a result of death, the children in affected families undergo severe psychological trauma before the death of their parents, as well as the continued suffering from maternal deprivation by infants who survive their mothers'. While expressed differently in different cultures, AIDS almost invariably has profound and disruptive effects on the family and the family structure.

Children orphaned by the AIDS epidemic need improved health, social and psychological services. They often need help from a variety of sources, such as schools, social work services, churches and the juvenile justice system (Nicholas and Abrams 1992; Ankrah 1993). A new social support network or compensating 'healing web' has to be established to meet this next wave in the AIDS epidemic.

Even if such an alternative social support network can be established, we have to be aware that the working-through process is complicated. Several authors (Moody and Moody 1991; Silverman et al 1992) have pointed to the fact that significant others often do not share in a communal representation of the deceased, and do not communicate with the children as the parent did, with all the little shared 'secrets', codes and non-verbal communication. A relative or friend that 'adopts' the child until the surviving parent is able to cope, may bolster the parent through his or her grief and may fill the immediate lack of parental emotional availability, but the parent's modeling of grief expression remains profound and significant. While adults invest their psychic energy in a variety of other people, roles and activities, young children invest almost all their emotional energy in their parents (Siegel et al 1990). To a certain extent, problems can be prevented if the parent(s) plan beforehand who is going to be the foster or adoptive parent. Many parents, however, do not plan for their children, which results from denial, fear of disclosure, lack of a potential guardian, or lack of planning capabilities (e.g. Giaquinto et al 1992; Nicholas and Abrams 1993; Ronald et al 1993). Children should be informed about the process, custody arrangements should be established, and even if the partner remains alive, children must progressively be prepared for the course of illness and death, in advance of deterioration (Lippmann et al 1993).

The lack of a potential guardian is a tremendous problem. Several authors have pointed to the fact that many of the children are taken care of by the grandparents, although this goes above their bearing power. Attention should be paid to this problem. Theoretically, the families of persons with AIDS (PWAs) include the nuclear and extended family and relatives, friends and lovers. However, many PWAs are estranged from family and turn elsewhere for support or totally lack social support. Driessen and colleagues (1991) showed that most of the injecting drug users that participated in a volunteer program had very small social support networks; most of the contacts were drug-related and could be characterized as instrumental.

Ultimately, the majority of HIV-affected children will end up in formal and informal foster care or adoptive care. Few of the programs that have been created to meet the needs of HIV-infected children, have also focused on the needs of HIV-affected children. Such programs are needed to train and supervise the future guardian to provide respite care, home assistance and other help in caring for HIV-affected children (Nicholas and Abrams 1992). The sooner this can be arranged, the better the chances that child and future foster/adoptive parent develop a communal experience of the deceased parent. However, it should not be forgotten that, although the adopted relative may fill the immediate lack of parental emotional availability, the parent's modeling of grief expression remains profound and significant (Moody and Moody 1991).

Addressing sickness, deterioration and death is not simple, however. It is relatively easier when a patient has entered the terminal stage (Siegel et al 1990; Christ et al 1991). With AIDS, there are additional obstacles to those communal with families where a parent dies from another disease. In addition to coping with the (upcoming) loss, families with AIDS have to deal with contagion anxiety, stigma, disclosure of 'secrets', such as betrayal over sexual orientation (e.g. bisexuality), extramarital affairs or former history of drug use (Lippmann et al 1993). Additionally, many of the families with AIDS fall into the categories of 'high-risk families' or 'vulnerable families' (Christ et al 1991). In many families, one or both of the parents qualify for a diagnosis of moderate or severe psychopathology, and enmeshed relationships are the rule rather than the exception. The presence of psychopathology and/or enmeshed social relations does not facilitate open communication on such issues as illness, deterioration, death, foster or adoptive care. If one of the major problems is to establish and engage in meaningful, lasting and reciprocal social relationships, building up a trusting, respectful and open relationship will be a most difficult effort, where more formal forms of psychotherapy are needed.

CONCLUDING REMARKS

Grieving children are not mini-adults. They present unique challenges because their responses to death are closely linked with developmental stages ranging from no understanding of death to a realistic view of death as part of life. In addition, working with grieving children requires an awareness of family dynamics and child development along with other factors precipitating dysfunctional grief. Children's parents are vital and influential role models. This means that children learn best to recognize, experience and express their natural emotions in supportive family environments, but it indicates as well that if a supporting environment is absent, then the coping abilities and development of a child are seriously taxed.

In cases of coping with the death of a parent, children usually mirror the type of coping style their surviving parent portrays. If the parent is able to address openly the death of his or her partner, this facilitates the expression of feelings, thoughts, beliefs and fantasies children have about the death. If the prevailing atmosphere created by the parent is one of not openly expressing emotion over the loss, other family members may conclude that revealing emotions to others is inappropriate and frightening. Feelings, fears and misconceptions cannot be addressed, with all possible detrimental consequences. Parents occupy a unique place in the center of the child's universe. While adults invest their psychic energy in a variety of other people, roles and activities, young children invest almost all their emotional energy in their parents (Furman 1964; cited in Siegel et al 1990).

In the Western world most HIV-infected and HIV-affected children stem from families that live in the poor areas of the developed world. Many of these families can be described as high-risk or vulnerable families. The level of structure, predictability and consistency is already low before HIV infection. After HIV infection, problems only increase. Thus risk impact is not reduced, but negative chain events follow instead. The sooner a supporting intervention in the course of HIV infection takes place, the better. Not only should the issue of guardianship and foster/adoptive care be addressed, it is equally important that this is done with respect to reproductive issues. Considering the negative impact of the death and the resulting almost unavoidable negative chain events, the decision to have children should be a fully informed and conscious one. It is for each individual to decide what degree of risk behavior he or she finds acceptable, but when others are involved in the consequences of risk-taking – that being the uninfected partner, or the uninfected or infected newborn child – dialogue is essential. The fact that so many newborns are abandoned immediately after they are born (Giaquinto et al 1992;

Nicholas and Abrams 1992; Ronald et al 1993), is indicative of impulsive and irresponsible decisive behavior. Ultimately, the choice remains with the parent; the counselor can facilitate discussion and make available information known (Goldman et al 1992).

Since familial background is a significant variable affecting children's grief reactions, working with children requires an awareness of family dynamics. Services must be set up which support the whole family structure and not parts as if they exist in isolation (Melvin and Sherr 1993; McGrath et al 1993). That is not to say that only family support should be delivered. On the contrary, there should be a continuum of services, offering individual counseling and support, mutual help and family support. Services, moreover, should include short-term activities supporting parents and children dealing with grief, as well as services that aim at ameliorating (pre-existing) intrapsychic and interpersonal psychopathology. Different services can have a synergistic effect. As an example, when parents become able to address their condition and its emotional impact in group or individual psychotherapy, they can often talk about it more readily with the family (Lipson 1993). However, the greatest challenge and the biggest problem is that those families that are in greatest need of help are the most reluctant in asking for it, and the most defensive if help is offered. Asking for help, unfortunately, is regarded as a sign of weakness, instead of as a sign of strength.

NOTE

1 Weinstein (1982, cited in Mireault and Bond, 1992) described perceived vulnerability to harm as an individual's perception of the likelihood of experiencing a threatening event. People tend toward optimism in evaluating their own vulnerability to negative life events. However, among individuals with personal experience of a negative event, the optimistic bias is reduced and perceived vulnerability to that or similar events is increased.

REFERENCES

Altschul S (1988) *Childhood Bereavement and Its Aftermath* Madison CT: International Universities Press

Ankrah EM (1993) The impact of HIV/AIDS on the family and other significant relationships: the African clan revisited *AIDS Care* 5: 5–22

Bergeron JP & Handley PR (1992) Bibliography on AIDS-related bereavement and grief *Death Stud* 16: 247–67

Van den Boom F, Gremmen T & Roozenburg H (1991) *AIDS: Leven Rond de Dood* Utrecht: Nederlands Centrum Geestelÿke Volksgezondheid

Caplan G (1990) Loss, stress, and mental health *Community Ment Health J* 26: 27–48

Christ GH, Siegel K, Palamera Mesagno F & Langosch D (1991) A preventive intervention program for bereaved children: problems of implementation *Am J Orthopsychiatry* **61**: 168–78

Demb J (1989) Clinical vignette: adolescent survivors of parents with AIDS *Family Systems Medicine* **7**(3): 339–43

Driessen A, van de Velden L, van den Boom F et al (1991) *Vrijwillige Hulpverlening aan Verslaafden met AIDS* Utrecht: Nederlands Centrum Geestelÿke Volksgezondheid

Furman RA (1964) A child's capacity for mourning. In EJ Anthony & C Koupernik (eds) *The child in his family: the impact of disease and death. Yearbook of the International Association of Child Psychiatry and Allied Professions Vol 2* New York: Wiley pp 225–31

Giaquinto C, Giacomet V, Pagliaro A et al (1992) Social care of children born to HIV-infected parents *Lancet* **339**: 189–90 (letter)

Goldman E, Miller R & Lee CA (1992) Counselling HIV positive haemophiliac men who wish to have children *Br M J* **304**: 829–30

Heagarty MC & Abrams EJ (1992) Caring for HIV-infected women and children *N Engl J Med* **326**: 887–8

Horowitz MJ (1986) Stress-response syndromes: a review of posttraumatic and adjustment disorder *Hosp Community Psychiatry* **37**: 241–9

Kane B (1979) Children's concept of death *J Gen Psychol* **130**: 141–53

Lippmann SB, James WA & Frierson RL (1993) AIDS and the family: implications for counselling *AIDS Care* **5**: 71–8

Lipson M (1993) Disclosure within families *AIDS Clin Care* **5**: 43–7

McGrath JW, Ankrah EM, Schumann DA et al (1993) AIDS and the urban family: its impact in Kampala, Uganda *AIDS Care* **5**: 55–70

Melvin D & Sherr L (1993) The child in the family – responding to AIDS and HIV *AIDS Care* **5**: 35–42

Michaels D & Levine C (1992) Estimates of the number of motherless youth orphaned by AIDS in the United States *JAMA* **268**: 3456–61

Mireault GC & Bond LA (1992) Parental death and parenthood: perceived vulnerability and adult depression and anxiety *Am J Orthopsychiatry* **61**: 517–24

Moody RA & Moody CP (1991) A family perspective: helping children acknowledge and express grief following the death of a parent *Death Stud* **15**: 587–602

Nicholas SW & Abrams EJ (1992) The 'silent' legacy of AIDS. Children who survive their parents and siblings *JAMA* **268**: 3478–9

Piaget J (1952) *The Origins of Intelligence in Children* New York: International Universities Press

Prichard S & Epting F (1991–1992) Children and death: new horizons in theory and measurement *Omega* **24**: 271–88

Ronald P, Robertson JM, Duncan JR et al (1993) Children of parents infected with HIV in Lothian *Br M J* **306**: 649–50

Rutter M (1975) *Helping Troubled Children* Harmondsworth: Penguin Books

Saler L & Skolnick N (1992) Childhood parental death and depression in adulthood: roles of surviving parent and family environment *Am J Orthopsychiatry* **62**: 504–15

Samperi F & Ahto L (1991) AIDS and survivorship: a three generational approach *I Int Conf Biopsychosocial Aspects of HIV Infection* (Amsterdam) Abstr 177

Siegel K, Palamara Mesagno F & Christ G (1990) A prevention program for bereaved children *Am J Orthopsychiatry* **60**: 168–75

Silverman PR & Worden JW (1992) Children's reactions in the early months after the death of a parent *Am J Orthopsychiatry* **62**: 93–104

Silverman PR, Nickman S & Worden JW (1992) Detachment revisited: the child's reconstruction of a dead parent *Am J Orthopsychiatry* **62**: 494–503

Tennant C (1988) Parental loss in childhood: its effect in adult life *Arch Gen Psychiatry* **45**: 1045–55

Tyhurst JS (1957) The role of transition states – including disasters in mental illness. In *Symposium on Preventive and Social Psychiatry* Washington DC: Walker Reed Army Institute of Research, Walker Reed Army Medical Center

Weinstein N (1982) Unrealistic optimism about susceptibility to health problems *J Behav Med* **5**: 441–60

Weller RA, Weller EB, Fristad MA & Bowes JM (1991) Depression in recently bereaved prepubertal children *Am J Psychiatry* **148**: 1536–40

Zambelli GC & DeRosa AP (1992) Bereavement support groups for school-age children: theory, intervention, and case-example *Am J Psychiatry* **62**: 484–93

CHAPTER 11

Death of a Partner: Responses to AIDS-Related Bereavement

Brigitte J. Richmond

University of New South Wales, Sydney, Australia

and

Michael W. Ross

University of Texas, Houston, USA

With the potential increase in deaths due to AIDS, an important area of growing concern is that of the psychological and social implications of the disease, especially bereavement. Of particular relevance is the understanding of features of bereavement that may be specific to AIDS-related deaths, along with the impact and distress of both the disease and the death on those who have close relationships with the infected person. An understanding and description of bereavement issues in relation to HIV infection would facilitate the development of appropriate forms of intervention aimed at reducing the level of psychological morbidity in those close to the person living with AIDS. This would also facilitate the development of effective and cogent models for training voluntary and professional services involved in providing counselling and other forms of psychological and psychiatric intervention in the AIDS area.

It is estimated by the National Centre for Epidemiology and Population Health that between 12 500 and 17 000 cases of infection with Human Immunodeficiency Virus (HIV) have been reported in Australia (Solomon, Fazekas de St Groth and Wilson 1990). From a total of 65 deaths from AIDS in Australia in 1985, there were 514 in 1992, with a cumulative total

Grief and AIDS. Edited by L. Sherr.
©1995 John Wiley & Sons Ltd.

of 2542 deaths by the end of 1992. Similar patterns are seen worldwide. It is apparent that AIDS-related bereavement is becoming an increasingly common phenomenon even outside the traditional epicentres of HIV disease.

PATTERNS OF BEREAVEMENT

Recent reviews of this field have emphasized the need for systematic research to examine patterns of bereavement in order to enable clearer clinical guidelines regarding the patterns of psychological symptoms occurring after the death of a partner. A number of reports have placed emphasis on the needs of the families of persons with AIDS and their partners, and in some cases have described cases of serious psychological disturbance in some circumstances, for example, suicide in parents and partners of HIV-infected persons (Holland and Tross 1985; Frierson and Lippmann 1988).

For those bereaved by AIDS, specific AIDS-related stresses may be experienced. For the partners, the risk factors for HIV are commonly present, as they may also be infected themselves and face the demands of coping not only with their own illness and possibly impending death, but also with the additional adversity of the loss of a loved one with the same illness. This poses a number of problems within the relationship, which are likely to complicate the bereavement.

These may include concerns about the source of infection in the couple, the needs for care of the more severely ill person, alteration in the quality of the relationship, plus a sense of watching what they will be going through (that is, a rehearsal of their own death). Additional losses such as friends becoming infected, loss of work with increasing illness and the stigma of the disease, may also impinge on the bereavement process. Further, the relationship may not be recognized by others as having the status of a primary attachment and therefore the recognition and acknowledgement of the partner's or family's grief may be diminished. Groups in the community most affected by HIV infection include gay men, people with haemophilia, and injecting drug users (IDUs). These groups may experience the deaths of a substantial number of their social network and the high exposure to death and threat to life may be sufficient to provoke post-traumatic reactions, such as may be found in other circumstances.

For family members the loss of an adult, child or sibling, may occur amidst ambivalent reactions to the infected person's sexuality or drug use. The often unexpected and untimely loss at this stage of an individual's life may result in excessive guilt and secrecy about the disease for fear of stigma by society. In many cases the family may also fear or experience the loss of social support and isolation if their own social support network becomes aware of the family member's diagnosis. Persons with HIV infection experience both loss and the psychological repercussions of these complex circumstances. A relevant dimension of bereavement is that of anticipatory bereavement, which refers to the process of reaction and adjustment to the anticipated loss, often in circumstances of protracted illness. Changes in close relationships and physical and intellectual deterioration are distressing and may accentuate the loss of the ill person prior to their death. Sowell and colleagues (1991) found from qualitative interviews that there were three themes occurring in a small series of AIDS-bereaved gay men. These themes were isolation and disconnections from family, lovers and self; emotional confusion (including guilt, anger, loneliness and ambivalence); and acceptance or denial of the loss.

Biller and Rice (1990) noted that gay bereavement was exacerbated by the coexisting issues of the stigmatization of both gay identity and AIDS, grief induced by repetitive loss, the lack of available biological family members, exclusion from involvement in funeral arrangements and lack of acknowledgement of the relationship between the bereaved and the deceased. There are no available data on IDUs in this regard, but it might be assumed that heterosexual IDUs and gay men would have strong similarities, as drug use is also heavily stigmatized. Indeed, several IDU respondents indicated informally that they were also stigmatized by the further implication that they were homo- or bisexual.

Geis, Fuller and Rush (1986), in an early study in 26 cases of the psychosocial stresses of being lovers of people with AIDS, found a number of responses. They found that there was strong evidence of societal stigma and isolation from friends, particularly social avoidance. A further pressure was the stigma from some religious sectors, associating AIDS with death and damnation, which was reported as being particularly hurtful and alienating, and which was mentioned by every interviewee. A third theme was 'passionate disrespect for the medical community'. Two particular areas of frustration were difficulty in diagnosis and continual changes in treatment protocol, as well as insensitivity to feelings on the part of some physicians. While Geis, Fuller and Rush recognized that the medical community usually bears the brunt of hostility when a patient's suffering and death cannot be avoided, painful experiences were noted, and most of the experiences with research teams were negative, with subjects resenting being treated as 'guinea-pigs'. Responses of biological families, these authors report, continued the themes of stigma, rejection and isolation – their requests for love and acceptance were met with varying degrees of disappointment. Attitudes toward the surviving lover's future were fatalism and obsession. A third, more rational response, was acceptance of the immunologic overload theory of AIDS and the belief that they could control the outcome. It is important to note that this study was carried out before the widespread availability of HIV testing and thus may be temporally biased.

Response to loss of a lover or close friend in New York City was studied in 1985 by Lennon, Martin and Dean (1990). They found in interviews with 180 gay men that the symptoms of grief observed were similar to those reported in bereaved spouses or parents. Intensity of the grief reactions was associated with a number of factors, the chief of which was having taken care of the lover or friend during the illness. Interestingly, the actual availability of instrumental and emotional support was unrelated to grief reactions, but the perceived adequacy of both instrumental and emotional support was strongly related to the level of grief. Those who had not received adequate caretaking support experienced more intense symptoms of grief than those who had received adequate support, with a similar pattern occurring for emotional support. These data confirm the similarity in response to losing a close friend or partner, regardless of the nature of the relationship, as well as the critical impact stigma and isolation may have through their impact on the perception of lack of practical and psychological support. However, the timing of this study is similar to that of Geis, Fuller and Rush, and the impact of stigma and isolation in 1985 may have been greater.

However, Martin (1988), in interviews with 745 gay men in New York, reported that 27% had been bereaved by AIDS, and of these, one-third had been multiply bereaved. Martin found a direct linear relationship between the number of bereavements and the symptoms of traumatic stress response, demoralization, sleep problems, sedative use, recreational drug use and use of psychological services because of AIDS-related concerns. That these findings were still strong after controlling for HIV status, symptoms of HIV disease and sexual behaviour history, suggests that these factors cannot explain these findings. It is of particular note that, because the symptoms of distress increase directly with the number of bereavements, there appears to be no adaptation to the continuing bereavements (at least, not up to the number (three) of bereavements that Martin studied). As Martin defined bereavement as being the loss of lovers and close friends, this parsimonious definition (close friends, he notes, are usually either former lovers or primary group members who function as a biological family to gay men) and its comparison with those who have lost friends or acquaintances probably understate the impact of bereavement.

COMMON THEMES

In a review of research into AIDS-related bereavement and grief, Bergeron and Handley (1992) summarized 43 works and found a number of commonly emerging themes. The 12 themes that emerged from studies of gay men surviving their male lover included: fear of having the virus (and going through what their lovers suffered); actually having the virus; lack of traditional recognition given to the survivor of a spouse in conjugal bereavement; lack of support through lack of community resources and support from family and friends; condemnation through the attribution of blame for infection or religious bigotry; and lack of closure through being excluded from funeral or memorial services. Other themes noted were conflict with lover's family or executor; survivor isolation (through people being too afraid to share their loss with others for fear of condemnation or exposure); internalized homophobia (self-blame for the loss because of anti-homosexual attitudes); lack of preparation for the death; the impact of multiple losses in the epidemic creating a bereavement overload; and fatigue and emotional and physical distress from caring for dying lovers. While these are not reported in all studies, they have been noted repeatedly and thus have considerable validity from being found in samples in widely varying times and places.

The progression of the HIV/AIDS epidemic means that more homosexual men and other groups at risk will experience bereavement. Many will experience multiple bereavements close in time. Thus, the epidemic is producing a situation in which grieving may become an unrelenting process with little opportunity for recovery (Lennon, Martin and Dean 1990). They found that gay bereavement was similar to that in other relationships, and was influenced by having taken care of the deceased, and adequacy of available social support.

PSYCHOLOGICAL DISTRESS

This chapter explores the existence of psychological distress among the families and partners of people who have died of AIDS, in order to provide a framework for its understanding. We intended to examine bereavement issues among the partners and families of HIV-infected individuals to increase our knowledge of the often hidden morbidity in those indirectly affected by the disease (Raphael 1986).

Data from a study carried out to explore some of these issues will highlight one of the concerns. Subjects were recruited from clinical sites in Sydney, through the cooperation of volunteer support agencies, social workers, advertisements in the gay media and through contacting other gay organizations (gay pubs, nightclubs, restaurants, day care centre, gyms and saunas). Participants were required to have a family member or partner who had died of AIDS, or to be living with the person with advanced HIV infection, requiring nursing or other supportive care at home or at specific community centres.

The total sample consisted of 16 respondents: 11 men and five women. There were substantially more bereaved men than women who had lost partners to AIDS, and more bereaved women than men who had lost family members. The mean age for women was 44 years and for men 40. The age range for both men and women was 27 to 57 years. The range of time since the death was 2 to 156 weeks, with a mean of 43 weeks. Because Lennon, Martin and Dean (1990) found that gay bereavement was similar to that in other relationships, we did not separate out the responses from those who had lost a family member and those who had lost a partner, although we emphasize the loss of a partner here. In most cases, there were few if any differences between bereavement situations in gay men and IDUs, but where these exist, they are noted.

The study included a questionnaire and a semistructured interview. This study reports only the open-ended questions as part of the face-to-face interview. The semistructured interview was conducted with each subject on a one-to-one basis, and lasted approximately 1 to 1.5 hours. All open-ended interviews were taped using a Dictaphone, and tapes were transcribed verbatim for analysis. This chapter reports on the transcript analysis of the open-ended questions. The main study and the Sydney cohort interview questionnaire modifications were approved by the relevant university ethics committees.

Positive Experiences with Bereavement

When respondents were asked whether they had any positive experiences with bereavement, some mentioned that they had developed useful survival mechanisms to help ease the suffering and pain, whilst others claim they relied on the strength and support provided by their friends and working colleagues. Positive experiences appeared to fall into the two categories of development of coping mechanisms and social support: friends very supportive and understanding ($n=4$, 25%); being able to cope with stress better ($n=4$, 25%); and being able to cope with the reality of death ($n=7$, 44%).

I have reached a spiritual plane that I never thought was obtainable. I actually know, beyond any doubt, that there are other ways of communicating, other than the physical.

Probably the best experiences I've had are with people from work, how accepting they were and how understanding they have been.

and from another respondent:

> The compassion, the unconditional love, support through friends and
> working with people who have AIDS, it's the most beautiful and important
> thing in my life so far. My life seems to blossom.

Respondents emphasized support received by friends and continually
praised professional help provided and support networks set up to help
them.

> I've got friends whenever I need them, who help to the best of their ability,
> I've been amazed at just how much support everybody has been.

It is interesting to compare this to findings in studies by Mount (1986)
and Raphael (1986). Their results suggest that sooner or later grief will
work itself out, and bereaved people will eventually stop grieving and
observe death in a more positive and objective light. They also state that
friends, family, support groups and professionals will help to lift the
weight and burden of grief off the bereaved. In this regard, AIDS
bereavement appears little different from other bereavement, as Lennon,
Martin and Dean (1990) also found.

How Bereavement Affected Survivor's Lives

Respondents described a barrage of varied and often conflicting emotional
states, when asked to describe how bereavement had affected their lives.
Although most individuals had accepted the death, they were still
confronted with problems socially, physically and professionally (noted by
$n=4$, 25%). Most described intense feelings of isolation or disconnection
which were associated with themes of loneliness, sadness and confusion
($n=7$, 44%). This seemed to be related to their inability to express their
feelings and thoughts with their families and at times with friends. Most
social support was gained from friends ($n=7$, 44%) and either
professionals or support groups (in each case $n=5$, 31%). Only one
individual nominated the family as a source of support. Others were angry
about losing family members and lovers who were so young and vital.
On the other hand, 32% ($n=5$) said that they had totally accepted the
death.

A sense of the effects of an AIDS-related bereavement can be gleaned
from the following accounts of men who have lost their lovers to the virus.

> I have had trouble with my anger, a lot of my feelings are caused because
> I feel lonely, shut off, and when I do start to express my thoughts I am
> often made, by others, to feel self-indulgent.

> I guess the things which have affected me are sadness and depression and times I wonder when it will all be over and there won't be any more people around me dying.

> I feel an incredible sense of loss that I can't seem to replace with any positive feelings. I'm so lonely I really find it hard to believe it is so final.

Studies carried out by Ross, Tebble and Viliunas (1989) with those diagnosed HIV-seropositive, and Kubler-Ross (1987) working with AIDS bereavement, support the above suggestions that withdrawal and depression are common symptoms found in those who are diagnosed with a potentially terminal illness. They concluded that individuals at this stage tend to keep to themselves, to fear infecting others, and that depression can arise through not being able to share the diagnosis. This reaction also appears to occur in the bereaved. Sowell and colleagues (1991) also noted this emotional confusion as a major dimension in the reactions of those bereaved by AIDS-related deaths.

Raphael (1986) suggested that 'to live is to experience loss'. She argues that losses do not occur in a vacuum, but interact with, modify and often augment the other stresses in both personal and professional lives. Further studies conducted in this area by Henderson and co-workers (1981), with regard to social support, and Biller and Rice (1990) and Lennon, Martin and Dean (1990), with regard to AIDS, found that the stigma surrounding AIDS and homosexuality can lead to homosexual men with AIDS being rejected by their biological family. There are no data on IDUs, but one might anticipate a similar response given the stigma which is also associated with drug use. Similar areas of research that focus on the effects of bereavement have been carried out by Lindy and colleagues (1983) and Raphael (1986). They found that anger and depression are ongoing, and often symptoms may increase in subjects who have suffered an impairment after a disaster as a result of bereavement or death experience. This may help the bereaved to protect themselves against the finality of loss.

Negative Experiences with Bereavement

When respondents were asked to share the worst experiences they had encountered with bereavement, most discussed varying degrees of loneliness, anger and ambivalence. Respondents who had watched their loved one die voiced deep feelings of anger and emptiness. Their anger seemed to be associated with the issue of 'why us?', as well as directed towards the deceased for leaving them to deal with their own vulnerability. The most common themes to emerge were feelings of emptiness and loneliness ($n=6$, 38%); watching someone you love die and dealing with the death ($n=6$, 38%); family (own and partner's) rejection ($n=4$, 25%);

not being able to talk about death and dying ($n = 2$, 13%); and employment problems ($n = 1$, 6%). Respondents also articulated feelings of anger at the lack of support and compassion shown by the families of both the deceased and the respondent during and following the death.

> I am angry and feel very let down by the way my lover's and my own family have treated us. I feel very isolated now that my lover has died and extremely confused about how I feel about life in general. Both families have abandoned us and now most of my friends have died, I feel very alone and disconnected from others.

> I wake up every morning and lay a place for my lover in the hope that he may return. Why does my life seem so empty? I have no direction anymore, I just live each day as it comes. Deep down I know that my lover will never return, but I can't seem to accept that it has happened to us. Why?

Raphael (1986) reported similar patterns of bereavement and found that the bereaved may often feel intense loneliness and emptiness due to the lack of acceptance of the individual's homosexuality by significant others. This desertion by the family may potentiate feelings of desertion or of loneliness from the death of the partner and exacerbate the loneliness or anger.

Research carried out by Biller and Rice (1990) suggests that the deceased is often the survivor's only real family, as the family of origin may be emotionally and geographically distant. Further, the family of origin and non-gay friends of the deceased may refuse to accept the survivor, causing a great sense of abandonment and isolation. This may also be the case with IDUs, as Stowe and co-workers (1993) have noted that non-biological family are often a greater source of social support than biological family in this group.

Most also felt that their own families had neglected their needs and as a result felt very isolated and disconnected from them. Individuals discussed the lack of compassion and sensitivity shown by their families, and believed that their families felt threatened by the fact that their son's lover had AIDS and the possibility that their son was at risk of infection. These reasons seemed to alienate the bereaved from their family. Over half ($n = 9$, 57%) said that they could not talk with their family about the bereavement (although five (31%) also reported being unable to discuss it with friends and three (19%) with work colleagues).

Studies carried out by Lindemann (1944), Raphael (1986), Singh and Raphael (1981) and Lindy and colleagues (1983) describe the feelings of powerlessness, loss, loneliness and despair felt by the bereaved. They gave similar evidence that the bereaved is often able to master death by talking through the death and loss. As the bereaved learn to live, survive, manage and have needs met without the deceased, they gain competence and confidence and their sense of mastery becomes more secure (Raphael 1986). However, the lack of involvement and compassion shown by the deceased's family in the final illness, often associated with lack of acceptance of their relative's sexuality or drug use, appears to differ in AIDS bereavement and may significantly exacerbate the distress. Biller and Rice (1990) noted that this may potentiate grief, and Lennon, Martin and Dean (1990) found that availability of social support reduced the impact of the grief reaction. The present data suggest that lack of family support may act in two ways: inducing anger at the lack of support and recognition, and lack of availability of support itself.

Memory of the Deceased

When respondents were asked to discuss experiences and memories shared with the deceased, individuals reminisced about the times they had shared, as well as the feelings and emotional strains and gains that they had experienced throughout their relationship.

> We had an enormously interesting life together, we discussed things together, we designed things together, travelled together, we had a thoroughly interesting and intelligent life together.

Others described attitudes and mannerisms that depicted the type of character the deceased represented.

> His advice to me prior to him becoming unwell – he was very much a mentor to me, I looked up to him for guidance, in decisions I made up about my life and it was almost like a co-dependent relationship. A lot of his attitudes have stuck in my mind.

The most common themes to emerge were holding on to memories and experiences ($n = 12$, 75%); the feelings they had for each other ($n = 10$, 63%), and in one case, the way they were treated by family and friends. Raphael's work (1986) supports those findings. She concluded that as there are many images and memories of the bereaved, there are likely to be many dreams. The bereaved may initially dream that the dead person is vividly alive and finds that each awakening is a painful renewal of grief. There is also a sense of happiness and reunion with such dreams.

> Sometimes when I wake up I feel that my lover is lying next to me and then when I look to see if it's just a dream, I frequently find myself becoming more depressed with each awakening.

> At times when I'm coming home from work I convince myself that my lover is waiting at home for me. Sometimes my dreams seem so realistic, it scares me.

Similarly, studies conducted by Volkan (1972) found that things that have belonged to the dead person may take on a special symbolic link with them, becoming linking objects. Raphael (1986) reported that when the bereaved is suffering from chronic grief, they may cry at every reminder, frequently visit the grave, hold conversations with the dead person and present all the hallmarks of unrelenting grief. In the present sample, there was no evidence of this although this may be due to the small sample number or sampling bias.

Funeral Service as a Focus of Distress

When asked to comment on the types of funeral services they had attended, the majority of gay respondents preferred gay funerals to the more structured and religious services. They explained that gay funerals represented a time to 'express one's individual relationship with the deceased'. They were seen as mostly happy and positive affairs, where friends and relatives joined together in a celebration for the deceased. Common themes regarding funerals were divided between positive and negative ones: 56% ($n=9$) saw services as positive and happy, but 25% ($n=4$) noted that funerals had been sad and depressing or conservative, religious and structured ($n=5$, 31%).

> My brother organized his own funeral, he played *The Wind Beneath My Wings* – that was for his lover because he believed that his lover was the wind beneath his wings – it was really beautiful. His friend had written a letter for my brother as the eulogy.

Those who attended more structured and religious services were frequently disappointed and often angered by the fact that the minister rarely acknowledged who the deceased was, their friends and the cause of death. The following example describes a more structured and religious service, depicted by one of the female respondents.

> When my sister died we weren't invited to the funeral by her husband, we weren't even told that my sister had died. We found out where the service was going to be held, and turned up. Her husband ordered one of the ushers to make us leave as it was a religious service, not a gay one.

A male interviewee reported:

> My lover's family shut us off. They refused to acknowledge that my lover was gay and had AIDS. When he died his family had a wake for him and claimed that he had died of cancer.

Biller and Rice (1990) found that before the actual death, partners had often been banned from seeing the deceased in hospitals and at home. Surviving partners are often excluded from the funeral plans and from attending the funeral.

Raphael (1986) has noted that the rituals of the funeral, the need to dispose of the deceased's possessions and to deal with unfinished business, all help the bereaved person to accept that the deceased has gone. Our findings point to the funeral in AIDS-related deaths as being an expression and focus of either the acceptance or rejection of the relationship (if it was a gay one) or of the deceased's sexuality (there were no comments regarding IDUs in our sample). Where this has been denied, the grieving process appears to take on a more traumatic quality.

> Making the funeral private and excluding me doesn't allow me to grieve, it denies or ignores the right to grieve.

While it might be anticipated that this would not be such a significant problem in heterosexual IDUs, we have no data to support or refute this speculation owing to the very small number of IDUs with AIDS in Australia.

Euthanasia

A second issue that arose was the response to euthanasia. Two respondents noted that the deceased had, in an advanced stage of illness, ended their life by drug overdose. These two expressed ambivalence, both about the fact that some people knew the circumstances (and a feeling that there was a stigma attached to it), and conflicting emotions.

> Euthanasia led to conflicting emotions compared to natural causes, and this jolted me out of my reaction to so many 'natural causes' AIDS deaths. My reaction was feeling cheated.

The same respondent also voiced concerns about euthanasia in relation to not being able to say goodbye, and to it being a truncation of an already shortened life where every moment was important. The tension seemed to arise between the intellectual acceptance of euthanasia and the emotional difficulty when it robbed one of time with the deceased.

Changes that have Occurred since the Bereavement

Following the death of a partner or a family member, most felt that they needed 'time out' to take control of the situation. They felt very emotionally labile ($n = 6$, 38%) and in some cases reluctant to have other relationships for fear of losing another lover to AIDS ($n=4$, 25%). Respondents wavered between feelings of guilt, anguish and ambiguity. Others felt they had established stronger ties with people and this was seen as a positive and personal gain. Other response themes fell into the categories of spending more time doing things on one's own ($n=6$, 38%) and being a lot closer to people ($n=3$, 19%).

> I enjoy time on my own. I have become a lot closer to some friends than I normally would have because I need people without consciously realizing it. I'm scared of having relationships, which makes it hard.

> I feel that since my wife has died I have spent a lot more time with friends that I normally would not have had time for. People that I thought were just acquaintances have really helped me through my trying period.

Kubler-Ross (1987) and Ross, Tebble and Viliunas (1989) found from their studies that withdrawal and isolation are very common symptoms in those diagnosed with both HIV and a terminal illness. Individuals tend to keep to themselves as part of their uncertainty of the reactions of others.

Raphael (1986) also found that the bereaved may lose their sense of purpose and withdraw from others. This may be due to others reminding the bereaved of the deceased, or because the bereaved is unable to go through the grief process with others faced with a similar situation.

Concerns about own Future with Regard to HIV/AIDS

When respondents were asked to describe the concerns they had with their future with regards to HIV, many ($n=7$, 44%) said they were not concerned. This was because they were in a monogamous relationship, had already contracted the virus and were not sexually active, practised safe sex or drug use, or had few sexual or injecting partners. Those who were worried about infection had either lost a lover to AIDS and believed that they were at risk of carrying the virus or were worried about having sex or sharing injection equipment without knowing their partner's HIV status. Paranoia about contagion was expressed by 19% ($n=3$), and 13% ($n=2$) said they were scared of having relationships. The same percentage said that they faced the reality of becoming ill and eventually dying. The following examples reflect the types of fears and issues faced by those interviewed.

> I am extremely concerned about myself and the possibilities of contagion. I don't have any more one-night stands, I'm really cautious about men and sex, it is a state of mind. I look at life in a different way.

> I often felt guilty that I had the luxury of a normal and healthy life whilst my lover was wasting away. I have tried to remain celibate at the fear of

contagion and I am also scared and I suppose I feel guilty in many ways, of entering into another relationship.

Flavin, Franklin and Francis (1986) reported that HIV might be used as a weapon to spread the illness through sexual activity, without precaution, warning or regard for others. These data suggest otherwise. The findings of Kubler-Ross (1987) and Ross, Tebble and Viliunas (1989) also support this, noting that a significant proportion of HIV-infected or bereaved people keep to themselves for fear of infecting others, with particular regard to HIV. Preoccupation with issues of reality, such as those of reinfection or infecting others, and the anticipation of punitive or rejecting responses, may also mask a neurotic acceptance of punishment, possibly stemming from internalized homophobia (or stigma associated with IDU: Ross and Darke 1992) in some cases.

Preparation for Bereavement

Individuals adopted various coping mechanisms to help prepare themselves for the death. Some ($n=3$, 19%) relied on the support and guidance of medical professionals and counsellors to progress through the grieving process. Others ($n=2$, 13%) were relieved when their loved ones eventually passed away for reasons referring to physical discomfort, diminished quality of life, and being unable to cope with watching the deceased suffer. Some individuals ($n=3$, 19%), however, were not prepared at all. They were aware of the programmes and support networks provided to assist them, but were unwilling to accept that the deceased was not coming back. The struggle to accept and cope with the death, was reflected in a statement given by a mother who had lost her son:

> I don't think that I prepared well for it at all. I mean, I was losing a son, how can one be prepared for that?

In some cases, it was the unreality of losing a child or person of the same age early in life that appeared to fall outside the conventional role of 'being bereaved', and led to lack of preparation. Thus, in addition to denial, the lack of models for some people was a difficulty. A quarter of people said it was 'just something you adapt to'.

Raphael (1986) examined inhibited grief, where the bereaved usually combines psychological numbing, overcontrol and containment of all feelings related to death. Respondents claimed that they had not experienced bereavement overload as such, but described multiple emotions in varying patterns. Others criticized the fact that support groups were predominantly constructed to cater for the homosexual sector of the community and that there were not enough heterosexual programmes established for people who had lost someone to AIDS. A significant proportion ($n=4$, 25%) said that they had not encountered any problems with bereavement overload.

Experience with Bereavement Overload

Kastenbaum (1977) coined the phrase 'bereavement overload' in reference to elderly people who experience many friends' deaths within a relatively short period of time. Leham and Russell (1985) apply this concept to those who deal with the multiple loss of persons with AIDS: 'Young adults are experiencing the loss of many friends within a few months or years. This is particularly devastating and frightening within the homosexual community'. Tyhurst (1951) had previously captured the sense of multiple loss in his study of acute disaster, where he suggested that a paradigm of three overlapping phases exists: the disaster; a recoil; and a post-traumatic stress period. Siegel and Hoefer (1981) and Di Angi (1982) suggest that loss reminds people of other losses; thus when gay people deal with the grief of someone dying, they are reminded of the grief of coming to terms with their own self-identity. In the present study, 32% ($n=5$) said that they had experienced bereavement overload, and 19% ($n=3$) said that they could not cope with the number of deaths they had experienced (although four (25%) stated that they had not experienced bereavement overload). One response was social withdrawal.

However, other issues occur to create or exacerbate bereavement overload. Several respondents suggested that such overload occurred by not being able to divide out one incident and express one's feelings about it. In addition, there was anticipatory grief for those still sick, and there was no sense of recovery, of its finite nature, or being able to achieve distance from it.

> I have certainly faced a substantial amount of bereavement overload because of the number of friends, including clients, who have died. It has affected me in that I have problems with my relationship. There does not seem to be a great deal of counsellors available, that is an area that needs to be looked into.

> When my mother and father died, I faced a tremendous amount of bereavement overload. Now that my husband is slowly dying of an AIDS-related illness these feelings are beginning to manifest.

> I haven't experienced any bereavement overload. I have been seeking counselling and my friends have been extremely supportive. I have been able to cope really well with the situation.

Biller and Rice (1990) found that for members of the gay and lesbian community, experiencing multiple loss of people with AIDS, the issue of resolving grief is complicated by society's inability and unwillingness to accept the gay identity, the importance of the loss of a gay significant other, and the consequent legitimate sense of loss the individual feels when a significant other dies from AIDS. In addition, the exacerbation of grief may be induced by repetitive loss over a limited period of time (what Lennon, Martin and Dean (1990) refer to as an 'unrelenting threat'). The present data suggest that AIDS bereavement overload, while containing elements of all these processes, may also be a function of the lack of finality and lack of a formal conclusion rather than the numbers or period.

CONCLUSIONS

The progression of the AIDS epidemic means that more homosexual men, other groups at risk, their families and their friends will become bereaved. Many of these individuals will continue to experience multiple bereavements close in time. Thus, the AIDS epidemic is producing a situation in which grieving may become an unrelenting process with little opportunity for recovery (Lennon, Martin and Dean 1990).

There are three significant aspects in which HIV infection differs from other terminal illnesses. First, HIV is not immediately terminal; secondly, it is usually superimposed on a stigmatized status associated with minority groups; and thirdly, there is considerable uncertainty as to the progression to terminal illness and uncertainty about the status of 'cures', vaccines or scientific breakthroughs, which are frequently discussed in the media.

Patterns observed in this study are consistent with similar studies conducted in this field. Specifically, family rejection or denial emerged repeatedly as a significant factor in bereavement, following the social stigma attached to both the diagnosis of AIDS and the homosexual or IDU life-style, and profoundly influenced the survivor's ability to progress through the grieving process (Sowell et al 1991). Support provided by friends and professionals was also a constant issue expressed by the subjects. Respondents wavered between feelings of loneliness, disconnectedness and isolation, which were associated with themes of anger, sadness and ambivalence.

Recent reviews of this field have emphasized the need for systematic research to examine patterns of bereavement so as to enable clearer clinical guidelines regarding the patterns of psychological symptoms occurring after death that are likely to indicate pathological grief and require specific intervention. A number of reports have placed emphasis on the needs of the families of persons with AIDS and their partners, and in some cases have described cases of serious pathological disturbances. Further, the recent works of Kubler-Ross (1987) on HIV infection provide little analytic discussion. Clinical experience also highlights the broad range of psycho-social problems encountered, which in many cases are best conceptualized as forms of adaptation to anticipated loss in the period prior to death and actual bereavement in the period following the death of the loved one. Application of the existing findings from the field of bereavement research emphasizes the high risk of morbid outcome for those experiencing such a loss.

Although the experiences of those studied are revealing, it is important to note that the respondents may not be fully representative of the broader targeted population. For example, considerable difficulty was encountered recruiting subjects who had just lost someone to an HIV/AIDS-related illness and there was also difficulty in obtaining subjects outside the metropolitan area of Sydney. Nor was it possible, given that the epidemic in Australia is primarily associated with homosexual men, to obtain a significant sample of IDUs and thus the representativeness of the IDU data from this sample is questionable. Further, the sample was small, self-selected, and biased toward the inner-city experience. For these reasons, we regard these data as suggestive for interventions and further research rather than definitive.

The specific findings of this exploratory qualitative study confirm many of the factors operating in bereavement that have been identified by previous researchers. It is not surprising that many of the features of bereavement found to apply to bereaved individuals also apply to those bereaved by AIDS. However, several probably unique variables also arose.

First, it was clear that grieving was ameliorated by social support, and the lack of social support because of the nature of the cause of death being socially stigmatized (or perceived as stigmatizing) did appear to lead to distress, as reported by Lennon, Martin and Dean (1990). Second, however, this appeared to be focused on the funeral ceremony as a hub of symbolism for the loss. If there was denial of the nature of the loss (through AIDS), or of the presence of friends, or the respondent's sexual orientation or drug use, then this inhibited grief and left the survivors unable to focus on the loss (the reality of which was denied). Where there was overt hostility from the biological family toward the survivor, this was exacerbated. Third, the more common occurrence of HIV/AIDS-related self-euthanasia provided a further element of tension between general beliefs about its appropriateness and the specific desire to hold on to the deceased as long as possible. Finally, bereavement overload appears to relate both to the number and temporal concentration of the occurrences of death from AIDS, and to its open-ended nature and the lack of a clear conclusion. This makes it an on-going rather than a past event. The clinical implications of this focus attention on the importance of allowing public ritual and recognition of grief and permitting closure. However, these findings are based on a small and unrepresentative sample and exploratory qualitative methods, and will need to be replicated in more extensive and quantitative, as well as clinical, studies. Nevertheless, the common themes that emerged are very similar to those reported by Bergeron and Handley (1992) and in other studies, which suggests that the process and content of grief in the loss of a partner have more commonalities than differences.

ACKNOWLEDGEMENTS

This study was carried out on the Sydney cohort of a larger study on AIDS-related bereavement awarded by the Commonwealth AIDS Research Grants Committee to Drs Brian Kelly, Michael Ross and Beverley Raphael. The contribution of Drs Kelly and Raphael to the literature review and the assistance of Ms Dixie Statham in coordinating the larger study are gratefully acknowledged. An earlier version of this chapter appeared in the *Journal of Psychosocial Oncology* (1994) **12**: 143–63 and is reproduced by permission of The Haworth Press.

REFERENCES

Bergeron JP & Handley PR (1992) Bibliography on AIDS-related bereavement and grief *Death Stud* **16**: 247–67

Biller R & Rice S (1990) Experiencing multiple loss of persons with AIDS: grief and bereavement issues *Health Soc Work* **15**: 283–90

Di Angi P (1982) Grieving and the acceptance of the homosexual identity *Issues Ment Health Nurs* **4**: 101–13

Frierson RJ & Lippmann SB (1988) Suicide and AIDS *Psychosomatics* **29**: 226–9

Flavin DK, Franklin JM & Francis RJ (1986) The acquired immune deficiency syndrome (AIDS) and suicidal behaviour in alcohol dependent homosexual men *Am J Psychiatry* **143**: 1440–2

Geis SB, Fuller RL & Rush J (1986) Lovers of AIDS victims: psychosocial stresses and counselling needs *Death Stud* **10**: 43–53

Henderson S, Byrne DJ & Duncan-Jones P (1981) *Neurosis and the Social Environment* Sydney: Academic Press

Holland JC & Tross S (1985) The psychosocial and neuropsychiatric sequelae of the Acquired Immune Deficiency Syndrome and related disorders *Ann Intern Med* **103**: 760–4

Kastenbaum RJ (1977) Death and development through the life span. In H Feigel (ed) *New Meaning of Life* New York: McGraw-Hill pp 35–47

Klein S & Fletcher W (1986) Gay grief: an examination of its uniqueness brought to light by the AIDS crisis *J Psychosoc Oncol* **4**(3): 15–25

Kubler-Ross E (1987) *AIDS: The Ultimate Challenge* New York: Macmillan

Leham V & Russell N (1985) Psychological and social issues of AIDS. In V Gong (ed) *Understanding AIDS* New Brunswick, NJ: Rutgers University Press pp 177–82

Lennon CL, Martin LJ & Dean L (1990) The influence of social support on AIDS-related grief reactions among gay men *Soc Sci Med* **31**: 477–84

Lindemann E (1944) Symptomatology and management of acute grief *Am J Psychiatry* **101**: 141

Lindy JD, Green BL, Grace M & Titchener J (1983) Psychotherapy with survivors of the Beverly Hills Supper Club Fire *Am J Psychother* **37**: 593–610

Martin JL (1988) Psychological consequences of AIDS-related bereavement among gay men *J Consult Clin Psychol* **56**: 856–62

Mount BM (1986) Dealing with our losses *J Clin Oncol* **4**: 1127–34

Raphael B (1986) *When Disaster Strikes: How Individuals and Communities Cope with Catastrophe* New York: Basic Books

Ross MW & Darke S (1992) Mad, bad and dangerous to know: dimensions and measurement of attitudes toward injecting drug users *Drug Alcohol Depend* **30**: 71–4

Ross MW, Tebble WEM & Viliunas D (1989) Staging of psychological reactions to HIV infection in asymptomatic homosexual men *J Psychol Hum Sexual* **2**: 93–104

Siegel RL & Hoefer D (1981) Bereavement counselling for gay individuals *Am J Psychother* **35**: 517–25

Singh B & Raphael B (1981) Postdisaster morbidity of the bereaved: a possible role for preventive psychiatry *J Nerv Ment Dis* **169**: 203–12

Solomon PJ, Fazekas de St Groth C & Wilson SR (1990) *Use of the Back Projection Method for Predictions of the Australian AIDS Epidemic* NCEPH Working Paper no 16. Canberra, Australia: National Centre for Epidemiology and Population Health p 33

Sowell RI, Bramlett MH, Gueldner SH, Gritzmacher D & Martin G (1991) The lived experience of survival and bereavement following the death of a lover from AIDS *Image: J Nurs Schol* **23**: 89–94

Stowe A, Ross MW, Wodak A, Thomas GV & Larson SA (1993) Significant relationships and social supports of injecting drug users and their implications for HIV/AIDS services *AIDS Care* **5**: 23–33

Tyhurst J (1951) Individual reactions to community disasters *Am J Psychiatry* **107**: 764–9

Volkan V (1972) The linking of objects of pathological mourners *Arch Gen Psychiatry* **27**: 215–21

CHAPTER 12

AIDS and the Death of a Child

Mary Reidy

University of Montreal, Montreal, Quebec, Canada

Children need to make sense of life and of the world around them, and death is an integral part of the world of a child in a family affected by HIV. However, children's perceptions, feelings, fantasies and fears about death are rarely communicated to the adults around them. We have some knowledge of the conceptualization of death in healthy children at various stages of development. We know little of the meaning of death or the significance of AIDS for children infected with HIV. To ignore their perception of death is to leave children prey to fears and anxieties; to be ignorant of their concept of death is to render questionable our attempts to care for them and to meet their needs (Wass 1984). The presence of AIDS particularly influences the way in which death presents itself: its inevitability is frequently confounded by the 'law of silence' which attends its presence (Reidy et al 1995). Moreover, infected children's experiences with loss, separation and bereavement may well add to their confusion and multiply their anxieties or affect their perceptions of death and dying.

MEANING OF DEATH, FEARS OF DEATH AND AIDS

The Concept of Death and Cognitive Development

The concept of death is acquired as part of a child's cognitive development within the experiential context of their sociocultural environment. While intelligence develops interactively with affect, theorists tend to focus on one or the other. Piaget (1973) postulates that children's reasoning is not just simpler or less detailed but is qualitatively different from that of adults and that their cognitive development leads, with maturity, to an adult cognitive structure. He divides cognitive development into life periods.

Grief and AIDS. Edited by L. Sherr.
©1995 John Wiley & Sons Ltd.

Nevertheless, the actual chronological age and rate at which children pass through the various stages of cognitive development, are not clearly differentiated in Piagetian theory. Common to all stages, however, is the progress from action to thought, from subjective to objective. As our current body of knowledge, theory development, research and intervention concerning death and children still rests in great part on these basic tenets of Piaget, it is important to keep them in mind when trying to understand the child affected by AIDS and death (Nagy 1948; Anthony 1972; Kane 1979; Guy 1993).

However, not only did Piaget (1973) concentrate on experience within an optimum childhood environment, but our knowledge of the significance of death in childhood also comes, for the most part, from research that has been carried out with healthy, non-bereaved children (Wass 1984). One can only expect differences between children who have experienced a parent's death, those who are themselves dying and non-bereaved non-dying children. Bowlby (1971a, 1971b, 1981), who has interpreted loss and separation in children in terms of developmental psychological theory, emphasizes the effect on growth and development of the child (including the development of the concept of death) with multiple and severe losses. This view is supported by Kastenbaum (1977), who maintains that in order to determine how any particular child interprets death, we must comprehend their developmental level, their personality, their patterns of communication and support and their life experiences. The HIV-positive child, particularly if s/he has been infected through vertical transmission, is likely to come from a family milieu that has been threatened by multiple losses, and whose members may be poor, socially alienated, have limited education or may be drug users and abusers (Boland and Conviser 1992).

Infants (0–2 years), Piaget believes, are unable to form concepts, but through repeated manipulation and exploration begin to discover that they are entities. For Piaget, a discussion of the meaning or significance of death for the child, at this stage of development, is inappropriate. However, by the age of 6 months, an infant perceives the difference between caretakers; and the delight and fascination with the game of 'peek-a-boo', at this early age, would seem to find its source in the intermittent thrill of the terror of separation (Hostler 1978; Maurer 1966).

Further, in studies and clinical observations of young children, Bowlby (1971a), Hug-Hellmuth (1965) and Anthony (1972) link death fears and anxiety with separation. Before the age of 2, the majority of children who are infected with HIV begin to experience separation and loss. The losses of these children can include loss of parent or sibling through death or hospitalization, separation or placement because of abandonment or excessive burden of care, loss of other significant nurturers or caregivers through changes in care routines, services or guardianship. The behaviour of infants who are HIV-positive, though they cannot express thoughts, fears and concerns verbally, provides information about their needs and their feelings. The effects of loss and illness are seen in their patterns of attachment to family and to replacement caregivers. They may seem overly dependent or withdrawn, to cry listlessly, and to be sad or to refuse to be comforted. Toddlers may experience difficulties in being with other children and in developing play skills (National Pediatric HIV Resource Center 1992; Viney et al 1992).

While certain anecdotal work indicates that children younger than 3 know about, but deny, death, other studies indicate that certain children, having experienced the loss of a loved one, can understand the finality of death at age 2 (Furman 1974). During this stage (2–7 years), rather than being able to define death, the child uses magical explanations. Death seems reversible or temporary, and the news of death may have little effect. However, the realization that a loved one will not return can be devastating. It is during this period that many children, suffering from AIDS, will die.

During middle childhood or pre-adolescence (7–11 or 12 years), children become conscious of their own subjectivity and of the distinction between their own thinking and the rest of the world. While the child begins to see death as irreversible, universal and personal during this period, it remains distant. Children tend to express concern and anxiety about the possibility of their own death. Concrete explanations are given for death. Early in the stage of development, accidents or disaster are seen as causes; later, natural causes such as illness and old age are added. The consequences and effects of death also become more logical in their minds: they talk of funeral arrangements, burial and decay. It is usually later, as an adolescent, that death is considered as an abstract.

Nevertheless, regardless of the very young child's ability to conceptualize death, both clinician and researcher are usually hard-pressed to comprehend the significance of the concept for the child because of the child's inability or unwillingness to verbalize. Still, those caring for the child infected with HIV through vertical transmission, must remain sensitive to the frequency and gravity of the separations generated by their disease process and that of their mother, to the basic fear of abandonment in the early stages of development, and to the effects of life situation and stress on conceptual development.

Meaning of Death and Fears of Death

Studies with healthy children, producing somewhat inconsistent results, indicate that children's beliefs, fears and concepts of death resemble those of their parents. These, in turn, are shaped by their religious beliefs, and their sociocultural environment (Lonetto 1980). Such beliefs and rituals may comfort, or may terrify if misunderstood or distorted by the immature child. Religious images of death may be compounded by television images, news documentaries and fiction. Conversations between adults about death and separation, stories and books provide further sources of learning. All are internalized and interpreted in terms of the child's level of maturation and ability to conceptualize (Wass and Cason 1984).

Humanist psychologists maintain that the impact of loss, such as death, is not as significant as the daily, continued interaction between child and nurturers (Combs, Richards and Richards 1976; Rogers 1991). Wass and Cason (1984), concurring with this view, point out that the cumulative sum of verbal and non-verbal communication between parent and child, convey worth, acceptance, approval or disapproval. Any fears that do develop can be stabilized in a milieu of clear communication and in an atmosphere of love. Research, based on this approach, does indicate that children's fears and anxieties about death are inversely related to self-concept and to the ability to manage such anxieties (Bluebond-Lagner 1977; Wass and Scott 1978).

However, mystery is part of the process of the growing consciousness which differentiates between internal and external reality. Everything possesses an element of mystery for the growing child: the changes in their body, their dreams, new words and concepts and adult conversations and actions. When their ignorance is accepted with empathy by their nurturers and their curiosity is rewarded, mystery resolves itself as they develop. Secrets can be imposed on the child either through the implicit actions and communications (or lack of communication) of the adults surrounding them, or explicitly through the imposition of a 'law of silence', as in the case of sexual abuse or infection with HIV. The child living with imposed secrecy is likely to feel shamed and to develop a lack of 'wanting to know', poor self-esteem and even psychological and psychosomatic pathology.

The secret of infection with HIV can become a pathological force which can drive the child into a quasi-insurmountable dilemma. On the one hand, they might be given information, by parent or nurturer, which clarifies communications with others but which they are compelled to keep secret. On the other hand, despite hints, clues and ambiguous messages, they may not be told the truth or most information is kept secret from them (Halprin 1993).

Death and the Significance of AIDS

Little seems to have been written about signification of death or of AIDS, or of the interrelationship between them, on the part of children with

HIV. However, studies carried out on the perceptions of healthy children, concerning disease causality (AIDS, colds and cancer) and awareness, knowledge and beliefs about AIDS, seem to support aspects of both the developmental and social learning theories about the conceptualization of death and dying. One study, representing the three major phases of cognitive development (7–9 years, 8–10 years, 11–13 years), indicates that children conceptualize AIDS in the same way that they do other diseases, which in turn reflects their cognitive development. However, despite the level of conceptualization, AIDS tends to be frequently linked with death and dying (Walsh and Bibace 1991). Other research (ages 9–11 years) indicates that children are likely to progress from viewing all diseases as more or less alike, with an undifferentiated causality, to the identification of more specific cause and differentiated risk factors. Nevertheless, while they tended to see cancer and AIDS as similar in that both could incapacitate and kill, they had more difficulty comprehending the difference in the contagious nature of the two diseases (Sigelman et al 1993).

Further, while many children were aware of AIDS by the first grade, all were aware by grade 6. Knowledge increased and misconceptions decreased with maturity. Nearly half of all children studied believed that someone they know will contact AIDS. More than three-quarters overall (50% in grade 1, 88% in grade 5) believed that most people with AIDS die. All tended to reflect some fear and anxiety about AIDS and people infected with AIDS. While few thought that the infected individual is to blame, they were about evenly divided on whether a person with AIDS could be a friend and if such a person should be isolated (Sly et al 1992). Other research with an analogous population reached similar results: 62% of first-graders had heard of AIDS and, by the end of primary school, not only had 90% heard of it but most possessed additional, if at times inaccurate, information (i.e. with respect to transmission). Most did not believe that a cure for AIDS existed and in discussing AIDS, or drawing pictures that represented AIDS, dying, death and symbols of death appeared with significant frequency (Fassler et al 1990).

While type and level of knowledge and fear of AIDS was found to increase with age in school children, preschool children indicated knowledge of the subject, being even cognizant of the concept of contagion (or 'catching'). Most of their knowledge of AIDS education seemed to come from the media, peers or school, with relatively little home involvement in AIDS education (Schvaneveldt, Lindauer and Young 1990). It would seem that parents' attitudes toward AIDS are associated with their children's attitudes, but not with their children's knowledge of AIDS. Children's knowledge, however, was a significant predictor of their attitudes. Most knew that AIDS was an incurable, fatal disease, most felt sorry for the infected person, that it was a big problem. Even so, nearly one-quarter felt that it happened to 'bad' people and as a punishment (McElreath and Roberts 1991).

The significance of AIDS and its association with death and dying among normal children is evident. If so, it may be postulated that the association is even more delineated for children infected with HIV who have experienced the death from AIDS of a parent or of another child at their treatment centre. An HIV-infected child may lose friends that they have made in clinic or even witness the death of friends in hospital units. Depending on the circumstances and the way in which the caregivers respond, assuming the child's lack of awareness, the inability to understand or the need to be protected from knowing may heighten the infected child's fears or multiply their misconceptions about death and dying (Boland and Conviser 1992).

ATTACHMENT, LOSS AND GRIEF

Attachment and Separation

The nuclear family (or variations of it), which remains the dominant family structure within the social context of Europe and North America, usually places the mother, for biological and cultural reasons, in the role of primary nurturer of the newborn. In fact, it is a widely held belief that a mother loves her child and the child loves his/her mother. Certainly, the infant bonds first and most intensively with her, then with surrogate nurturers who, in most cultures, are the father or other members of the extended family, such as the grandmother. The child is far from passive in this process and the sensorial capacities of even the newborn allow interaction with those with whom he/she comes in contact. Such interactions, even with surrogate caregivers, can generate communication and attachment (Bourdeau 1986; Bourdeau and Taggart 1995).

Bowlby (1971a), in his momentous work on mother–child attachment, discusses the dynamic equilibrium between, on the one hand, the child's attachment behaviour and behaviour which is antithetic to attachment, and on the other, the mother's caretaking behaviour and her behaviour which is antithetic to parental care. The latter includes behaviour that competes with child care for time and energy, such as work or care of her own health. However, certain maternal behaviour, such as withdrawing from the child because of the burden of care or expressing dislike or disinterest in the child, is inherently incompatible with infant care.

In bonding, nearness and interchange are pleasurable to both, separation and rejection are disagreeable and even painful. During the course of childhood, the responsibility for maintaining proximity shifts progressively from mother to child. Various conditions 'activate' the attachment behaviour of the child, influencing its form and intensity. These include the condition of the child (i.e. hunger, illness, pain, etc.), the behaviour of the mother (i.e. absence, illness, rejection, etc.) and other environmental conditions such as alarming events (i.e. bright lights, hospitalization, treatments, strange noises, etc.) or rebuffs by other adults or children (i.e. scolding by health professionals, teasing or hostility by peers, etc.). With time, the normal process of separation takes place. Attachment behaviour becomes less frequent and less intense as the infant matures during childhood, adolescence and adulthood, encountering a great variety of social interactions. Attachment to parents is usually reduced in intensity through the 'normal' process of separation, though contact is maintained or even terminated as other social relations predominate.

Separation, however, that is premature contains elements of ongoing powerlessness, frustrated hope and rejection and provokes feelings of loss and bereavement. The equilibrium of behaviours in the mother–child dyad is severely threatened when the mother or both the mother and child have AIDS. The neonate of an addicted mother or the child who becomes symptomatic in the first year of life, because of spasticity, pain, central nervous involvement, iatrogenic treatment effects or irritability, may be slow to show attachment behaviours such as smiling or reaching for the mother or surrogate caregiver. The child may frequently show behaviour antithetic to attachment, such as inconsolable crying, withdrawal or tantrums (Anderson and Emery 1990).

The mother, who is HIV-positive or even symptomatic, frequently retains her role of homemaker and often that of breadwinner. If she is symptomatic or being followed and treated prophylactically, she must visit doctors and even submit to hospitalizations. She often assumes the role of primary health care agent for herself, her child and even her spouse. On the one hand, all of these behaviours not only compete in time with maternal caretaking behaviours but they are being performed by a mother subject to a disease process that produces fatigue and drains energy (Reidy et al 1995). On the other hand, absence, emotional withdrawal, depression, anger, neglect and abuse are behaviours antithetic to the attachment process. Because of her own state of health, drug addiction, guilt over the child's infection, shame, stigma, or fear of her own or her child's death, she may behave in ways which are not intrinsically compatible with bonding.

Why do women who know that they are infected with HIV become pregnant and give birth to children? Is it despite the fact that they themselves are going to die, or is it, in fact, because these mothers realize that they are going to die? The decision to have a child is the inevitable outcome of many conflicting forces in their lives. Cultures, subcultures and even individuals who are alienated or feel themselves threatened tend to seek affirmation of life and hope for the future in reproduction (Boyd-Franklin and Aleman 1990). Certain cultures equating love with reproduction, see a child as the necessary product of a committed love relationship. Women with other chronic diseases who give birth to babies at risk to themselves, are usually admired by society. However, HIV-positive mothers are frequently looked upon as being irresponsible for having babies who will die or become a burden to the community (Levine and Dubler 1990).

While less than one-quarter of HIV-infected mothers give birth to babies who prove subsequently to be infected, seropositivity in the newborn remains an indication of the mother's HIV infection status rather than of the child's actual infection (Mock et al 1987). While rates vary from study to study, it would seem that approximately 15% of infants, seropositive at birth, are admitted to hospital (one to eight times) with AIDS-related diagnoses within 12 months of birth. Over 20% of these infants die during these hospitalizations. Hope and uncertainty play a part not only in the process of attachment between these infants and their mothers or surrogate caregivers but also in the bonding dyad (child–nurturer) of the other infants whose infection status may not be confirmed until after 18 months of age (Gelbatis, Novik and Stacy 1991). While the effects of maternal deprivation can be devastating to the newborn, discordance in the mother–child relationship can also disrupt the bonding process. In fact, failure to thrive from birth in certain of these infants may not be due only to the pathological effects of the illness but may also be a function of separation and loss.

The 'normality' of the process of separation in the mother–child or the adaptation to other losses depends, in part, on the maturity of the child and on the quality of surrogate nurturance. The most common replacement or permanent surrogate caregivers of children who are orphaned or whose parents are no longer able to care for them because of HIV infection, are other family members. Grandmothers, with whom the children have already formed an attachment, frequently fill this role. However, as nurturers, foster parents are committed to a process of attachment with a child who is already probably bereaved and who most certainly will die within a fairly short span of time. However, while predictable or even imminent death of the child does not necessarily impede or distort the attachment process, a surrogate caregiver must give a great deal of herself or himself in order to accomplish the particular type of bonding involved in the support of the dying child (American Academy of Pediatrics 1989; Meintz and Lynch 1989; Sherr 1991).

Loss and Bereavement

Bereavement is a state of being bereft and feeling sad following the loss of someone or something. Partial losses such as the loss of bodily closeness of the mother–child relationship, loss of favourite toys or clothes or the skills of dressing, and the loss of separation, such as during a hospitalization, are not total and final as is the loss of death. Nevertheless, their effect on the child, under certain circumstances, can be as profound: they change what the child is, what they have and how they see themselves (Furman 1984). The child with AIDS poses a very special problem. In many instances, there is social stigma and isolation associated with the diagnosis and, in addition, the child is from a family in which the mother, among other family members, is also infected. The child, then, may be bereaved even as they die (Reidy, Taggart and Asselin 1991; Sherr 1991).

Green and Sherr (1989) discuss the spectrum of losses of adults infected with HIV, which go beyond those associated with the imminence of death. Many of these are also felt by infected children. There is a loss of health with an incumbent restriction in the normal activities of childhood, as well as changes in life-style brought about by deterioration in the standard of living or conditions of living of infected parents. Feelings of certainty, about what will happen tomorrow or next month, and sentiments of control of immediate situations, or even body control, disappear as the disease evolves progressively and erratically, and treatment demands increase. Children, just as adults, suffer from the loss of privacy and dignity associated with extensive tests and invasive interventions. They also suffer from losses concerning body image, in how they feel about themselves and how they think others see them. Their social relationships can be threatened because they are infected by HIV. They can be abandoned by family members, shunned by neighbourhood children and even refused entry into school and day-care programmes. Older children and adolescents can suffer the loss of hopes for the future: what they might have or experience as children or what they might do or become as adults, as well as the hope for romantic love, sexual development and children of their own.

Children's reactions to bereavement include behavioural symptoms, psychological distress and physical problems. They may experience shock, guilt, depression and anxiety. They may become angry as they realize the extent of their loss or are unable to comprehend the events that surround the loss. They are curious and ask questions that perplex or threaten adults. Moreover, while young children feel pain and grief, they may not manifest them in the same behaviours or at the same rhythm as an adult. They play, laugh and smile; outward manifestations of mood do not necessarily reflect the loss or the trauma of the loss that they are experiencing (Sherr 1991).

Grief and the Work of Grieving

The term 'mourning' is often used in the narrow sense, as a synonym for 'grief', representing the painful, emotional aspects of loss. Conceptually and clinically, it would seem to be more appropriate to apply the concept of mourning to a wider variety of mental states associated with loss and to the concurrent cognitive work following the loss of a loved one to death (Furman 1984). Normal mourning is seen as a process of internalization of the qualities of the deceased and the coming to terms with their faults: the return to a reality where new attachments are possible. It is a psychosocial transaction whereby the individual experiences a major change and is led to reconstruct their perception of the universe as well as their place in it. Mourning, as it evolves, can become an occasion of growth and transcendence of self with a reconstruction of self with new rules, other values and different attitudes and behaviour. However, various pathological mourning processes can and do occur. They include: chronic mourning (it seems that it will never end); delayed mourning (it only appears long after the event); exaggerated mourning (it is amplified to the point that the mourner becomes dysfunctional); and masked mourning (it appears later in the form of physical or psychiatric symptoms) (Bacqué 1992; Parkes 1979; Penson 1990; Worden 1991; Fontaine and Reidy 1995).

Many authors conceptualize mourning as steps or phases in a process. Despite the danger of stereotyping adaptive behaviour in the face of death and of ignoring the holistic nature of the grief process, this conceptualization can be helpful to clinician and researchers, as well as to those who grieve, if the relative nature of the process is kept in mind (Corr 1992). A well known example of the process is found in the work of Kubler-Ross (1969, 1983) who speaks of stages of denial and isolation, anger, bargaining, depression and acceptance. More recently Monbourquette (1992) has added three steps to this sequence: pardon – permitting the liberation of anger and guilt; 'letting-go' – a form of goodbye; and psychic inheritance – allowing the recuperation of memories of the loved one.

The death of a parent, the primary nurturer, is certainly the most significant loss a child can experience, creating an immediate crisis or trauma with long-lasting effects on the child's mental health (McCown 1988; Parry and Thornwall 1992). In his studies on separation and loss, Bowlby (1981) has observed in children more than in adults, a preliminary phase, a type of shock whereby the bereaved child is completely overcome. They are astonished and seem incapable of accepting the news:

the denial of the reality of the loss becomes the primary reflex in response to the loss. Little by little denial gives way to anger, and intense distress is replaced by listlessness and longing, followed by disorganization and despair. This latter phase permits the evolution of mourning toward the final phase of reorganization when life is resumed and the mourner adapts to their new situation. The biological function of grief (i.e. to regain proximity to the attachment figure) cannot be realized in the case of death. The child, according to Bowlby (1971b, 1981), avoids dysfunctionality if they are actively able to work through their loss and redefine self in terms of the changes that have occurred in their life.

Earlier bereavement can help or hinder the resolution of current grief, as the latter is tributary to the former. First death experiences in childhood are important in how one sees life and subsequently death. Parents or other caregivers are at times hesitant, or forget, to include children in death rites and rituals. How a child is treated, not being permitted to cry, to express sadness or to talk about death or the person (or even the pet) who has died makes it more difficult to cope with later experiences of death. The use of unrealistic euphemisms such as 'merely sleeping' or 'gone away' can lead to sleep disturbances and anxieties (Dyregrov 1991; Dickinson 1992).

Children infected with HIV are exposed to many factors that can facilitate, complicate or disrupt the normal process of mourning (Abrams and Nicholas 1990). The nature and the strength of the attachment between the child and the dying parent are primary. However, the stigma of death from AIDS and the presence of the associated phenomenon of multiple losses can also complicate the resolution of mourning. Age, sex, tolerance for suffering and anxiety, the capacity to express feelings and the quality of substitute nurturing, as well as belonging to a religious or cultural group with attendant ritual, imagery and symbolism, can also influence the grief response. Furthermore, social factors associated with HIV infection (i.e. social negation or rejection, imposed silence, social or geographical isolation, or the need to assume the role of 'super strong'), are seen as contributing to a pathological grief process (Rando 1984; Worden 1991).

Children are in the power of adults because of their basic and psychosocial needs and because of the adults' control of information. Preventing or distorting the flow of information is often done, in the child's 'best interest', in order to prevent pain or to protect them. Such decisions result in a conspiracy of silence which may deny the child the information required to 'make sense' of the loss. If they do not know, they can only imagine (Jewett 1982). Moreover, Bowlby (1981) indicates that children will grieve and eventually resolve their loss if they have a secure relationship with their primary nurturers, receive accurate and appropriately conveyed information, are allowed to ask questions and to participate in the family grieving process, and have a surrogate nurturer on whom they can rely for a continuing relationship.

The 'grief work' hypothesis states that coping with grief, which prevents lasting health consequences, implies a process of confronting one's loss or of bringing the reality of the loss into one's awareness. This hypothesis, which has become a firmly entrenched belief in Western clinical practice, serves as the basis of many therapeutic interventions that share the common goal of facilitating grief work. Stroebe (1992–1993) questions the hypothesis, both on the lack of empirical data and on crosscultural evidence. Few experimental studies seem to support the hypothesis as it is currently formulated, and documented reports of reactions and customs seem to indicate that, within certain cultures, it seems more beneficial to restrain or suppress grieving rather than to confront the loss. While grief work intervention would seem to be most appropriate in the context of pathological grief, she proposes, even in this context, a reformulation that excludes rumination and expression of negative affect. Grief work, in this more restrained reformulation, is seen as a confrontational cognitive process that involves restructurization of the thoughts of the bereaved about the deceased, their experience of loss and their changed life-situation.

THE DYING CHILD

The Clinical Picture of the Child in the Terminal Phase of AIDS

In order to understand the dying child with AIDS, one must comprehend the physical ravages of the abnormal physiological and pathological effects of HIV infection, of opportunistic and secondary infections and of the side and untoward effects of medical regimens (Pizzo and Wilfert 1991; Boland and Conviser 1992). In the early stage of HIV infection, the child becomes susceptible to recurrent bacterial (particularly Gram-positive) and fungal skin infections; skin and mucosal infections follow bites, eczema and catheter insertion. They become subject to common skin infections including cellulitis and abscess infection, to frequent sinopulmonary infections including pneumonia, sinusitis and otitis media and others such as influenza or staphylococcus. They are also likely to suffer from various gastrointestinal infections, including salmonella.

As the disease progresses, various infectious agents which usually present little threat to the individual with a healthy immune system, invade the immunocompromised child (Hauger and Powell 1990). The most common of these so-called opportunistic infections include:

Pneumocystis carinii pneumonia (PCP), *Candida esophagitis* (recalcitrant oral thrush), cytomegalovirus (CMV), *Mycobacterium avium-intracellulare* (MAI), *Cryptococcus meningitidis*, toxoplasmosis and cryptosporidiosis. Central nervous system (CNS) disorders are also of great concern in these children. Further, while malignancies appear much less often in children than in adults, certain paediatric cases of Kaposi's sarcoma and B- and T-cell lymphomas have been identified (McClain and Rosenblett 1990). Because of the prolonged survival time of infected children attendant on improved treatment, increased incidence of malignancies is to be expected.

The child with advanced AIDS will present singular or multiorgan system involvement (Wiznia and Nicholas 1990). The respiratory tract can be compromised by lymphoid interstitial pneumonitis (LIP) with related hyperplasia of bronchus-associated lymphoid tissue leading to dyspnoea and hypoxaemia. Gastrointestinal tract disorders, such as diarrhoea and vomiting, have both common causes as well as condition-specific aetiologies such as CMV and retrovirus gastroenteritis.

Developmental delay, a frequent sign in HIV-infected children, can be compounded by the *in utero* effects of maternal drug abuse or by congenital syphilis, which produces CNS involvement. Other indications of CNS involvement include seizures, ataxia, abnormal tone, spasticity, corticospinal tract degeneration and acquired microcephaly. Encephalopathy can be progressive or static. Encephalitis, meningitis and retinitis, CNS disorders of great concern in these children, can be caused by herpes simplex, varicella zoster or Epstein–Barr viruses.

These children also suffer from haematologic disease, renal complications and cardiomyopathy. Most haematologic disease in HIV-infected children results from an increased rate of platelet destruction. Moderate or severe anaemia and thrombocytopenia may be present. The disease process may be caused directly by the HIV infection, or result as a secondary effect of being immunocompromised or as side-effects of drug intervention. Moreover, while these children suffer less often from nephropathy and from renal failure leading to death than adults, they are found to suffer from focal glomerulosclerosis, mesangial hyperplasia and infiltration of the kidney by B- and T-cell lymphomas. Finally, while the primary or secondary nature of cardiomyopathy is uncertain, some children have been known to develop congestive heart failure with pulmonary oedema, tachycardia and decreased peripheral pulse.

The most common medications used to treat this myriad of disease processes, signs and symptoms, tend to be fairly new or experimental, costly and to have many untoward side-effects. These drugs include: AZT (Wellcome) (zidovudine), dideoxycytidine, dideoxyinosine, acyclovir (Zovirax), amphotericin B, 5-fluorocytosine, trimethoprim–

sulfamethoxazole (TMP–SMX), pentamidine isethionate, ganciclovir, nystatin (mycostatin), ketoconazole and steroids (prednisone and others). Recorded side and iatrogenic effects of these drugs include: gastrointestinal upset, vomiting, diarrhoea, constipation, fluid retention, skin rash, fever, chills, hypoglycaemia, pruritus, neutropenia, anaemia, hypotension, interstitial nephritis, potential liver toxicity, renal toxicity, electrolyte imbalance, bone marrow depression, nausea, severe enterocolitis and hepatotoxicity (Boland and Conviser 1992).

The presenting clinical picture, in the terminal phase of AIDS, is that of a child with an increased susceptibility to infections who frequently suffers from fever and possibly chills. They have a potential for bleeding and for impairment of skin integrity. They most probably suffer from an alteration in gas exchange and in fluid and electrolyte balance, which is intensified by diarrhoea or vomiting, and they have probably lost weight. Suffering from wasting syndrome, they have an increased nutritional need for ingestible and absorbable proteins and carbohydrates. However, possibly because of thrush, mucosal ulcers of the mouth, throat or oesophagus or because of nausea, lack of appetite, unfamiliar or unappetizing nutrients or emotional withdrawal, they are reluctant to eat. They may react to their illness and treatments with depression, anger, fear, shame or confusion. Sleep patterns will probably be disturbed and they may well experience increased night-time activity. As the disease progresses, they will develop an increased need for pain and symptom management (Daily 1991).

The Dying Child's Awareness of Death and Fears of Dying

Everyone is afraid of death when children are dying: the children themselves, parents, siblings, nurses, doctors and social workers. Children who are gravely ill are concerned about dying. While they want to talk about it, their environment frequently discourages even questions. Seriously ill young patients sense what is happening even when attempts are made to shield them from a frightening situation. Even very young children present evidence of awareness of their illness and their approaching death, through their behaviour and symbolic questioning (Binger et al 1969; Kubler-Ross 1969, 1983; Waechter 1984). In a study of four groups of chronically ill children, intensity of treatment (paralleling exacerbations in the evolution of the disease process) was found to be the most significant factor in the production of death imagery in their stories (Waechter et al 1986).

It was maintained during the 1950s and 1960s that, because of their level of maturity, children with fatal illness would be harmed by dealing with their feelings about death. Parents were encouraged to shield children from knowledge of serious illness and approaching death. This approach gave way to controversy, based on the belief that the parent's burden of silence would cause withdrawal and lack of trust on the part of the child, who would have learned not to ask disturbing questions. However, Sherr (1991) in discussing the death of children with AIDS, maintains that, even now, silence, denial and pretence are often present when a child is dying. Overtly or symbolically, the child and their family have the need to say farewell: the dying child should, like an adult, have the right to know and be given the opportunity to plan.

In a study of children (6–10 years) with life-threatening illnesses, Waechter (1971) found not only a great dichotomy between their awareness of their prognosis and parental belief in this awareness, but also an inverse correlation between the opportunity to discuss their fears and specific death anxieties. Their caregivers, family and professional, seemed blinded to such awareness by their own fears. In a later study with parents of children of the same age group, Waechter (1984) found that most parents felt that they should be open with their children and answer their questions. Most discussed treatment; however, the younger the child, the less prognosis was discussed. Terminally ill children recognize that they are dying through a prolonged process of acquisition and assimilation of information, well before death is imminent. Bluebond-Lagner (1989) refers to this process as 'internalization' when they are told about their diagnosis and prognosis and their questions are answered openly and as 'discovery' when the children are not told. In either case, children gather information from the behaviour and reactions of others and from their own response to the disease process. They pass through various stages, from realizing that they have a serious illness to a view of themselves dying, in a cumulative process of collecting information. Their behaviour in the final stage reflects their view of death, which may be internally contradictory. This view, which will reflect their stage of developmental maturity, may well represent a model of children's view of death that is different from that of healthy children (Bluebond-Lagner 1989).

Lipson (1993) asks: 'When a child is dying of AIDS, what can she understand and what can her parents bear to tell her?' Rarely do AIDS parents wish to relate the prognosis or the details of their illness to children under 4 years old. By the age of 14, however, few parents doubt that the adolescent must be told. Between these two lies conflict and doubt. In Lipson's experience (1993), most school-age children are not told of their diagnosis. When a parent says that a child is not old enough to know, they may mean that the child cannot understand the aetiology of HIV, that they cannot keep the diagnosis secret or that they are not capable of understanding death.

Parents and caregivers have reason to fear the disclosure of AIDS and to face the subsequent discussion of death with reluctance. Their experience on hearing their own or the child's diagnosis was probably painful. Children, even with HIV, are loved and are often the family's hope for the future. To discuss a fatal disease is to invite death into consciousness. Disclosure, it seems, might even cause the child to get sick and die sooner. Disclosure also means discussing the parent's illness, guilt and death and coming to terms with ostracism if the child tells others. Further, strategies of vulnerable minority or alienated groups, for coping with threat of loss, usually include avoidance rather than openness. Perhaps the reasons for non-disclosure of most parents are based on self-interest or non-adaptive caring strategies, but whatever harms the caregiver in this fragile child–parent relationship will certainly have an effect on the well-being of the child.

The Dying Child's Way of Coping with Death and Dying

Young children with life-threatening illness such as AIDS, suffer threat to body image just at the time when healthy children are mastering motor skills, and becoming comfortable with their bodies. They may see flaws in their bodies, such as extreme thinness, or experience the loss of acquired motor skills such as walking or dressing, during acute exacerbations of the illness. Having developed only immature concepts of causality, preschool children tend to find the cause of illness in their own behaviour, often as punishment for misdeeds or even evil thoughts. They are also incapable of seeing the causal relationship between illness and treatments and the pain they cause. Severely ill and dying children cannot recognize the therapeutic intent of health professionals when interventions are seen as punishments. Unable to express anger and resentment openly, these children often become withdrawn or aggressive. Their fears of death can become attached to the cycle of guilt and punishment. At the age of 4, as discussed above, many children are conscious that death occurs, and may see their death as part of a continuing process of retribution. They fear being left alone to die and some who have developed religious concepts, even fear not going to heaven (Waechter 1984).

The school-age child is better able to cope with threat, even that of a terminal illness. They are beginning to understand cause and effect and can solve problems with thought as well as by action. In Waechter's study (1971), almost all school-age children with leukaemia asked questions about the future, some by direct questions, others obliquely. Because of increasing survival rates, in recent years, of children suffering from various fatal childhood chronic diseases (even AIDS), school becomes important, not only for the development of social relationships, but also as preparation for an uncertain future. However, the child with AIDS adds stigma and social isolation to the problem of peer relations, made difficult by frequent absences because of illness and hospitalizations. Body image assumes an even greater importance with increased peer involvement. Loss of weight, bruises from injection sites and other marks or signs of illness can be a source of distress for the infected child and a source of discrimination from peers. It is also likely that children with AIDS, because of decreased growth and development during acute phases of the illness, resemble children with cancer in that, compared with healthy children, they have difficulty in initiating or participating in activities.

School-aged chronically ill children, like other healthy children, tend to become more independent from their families as they mature. Nevertheless, as they move into the terminal phase of the illness, they become frightened of the pain, aware of death and dying and often hostile towards treatments and the treatment team. Many of the children in Waechter's study also question why they had been singled out for this illness, the feelings of guilt and punishment being less important than in younger children but still evident. A sense of trust and a feeling of support as well as knowledge about their condition and the ability to exercise control in the situation were all required by these children in order to cope with the stress of the terminal phase of their illness. A later study of children with cancer confirmed that an open communication pattern was closely associated with successful coping (Spinetta and Malony 1975).

The Social and Familial Context of the Child in the Terminal Phase of AIDS

'Normal' family life and effective parenting (by whoever assumes the role) may be hampered by the impact of AIDS on the family. Family members may suffer social and emotional isolation because of ostracism or may practise the 'law of silence' in order to protect the family. This self-imposed secrecy may include: refusing to seek community support for fear of revealing their diagnosis, hiding the diagnosis in social relationships, from schools and from social agencies, or 'covering up' the circumstances of the illness or death of a family member (Murphy and Perry 1989; Daily 1991; Melvin and Sherr 1993; Reidy et al 1995).

The fatal illness of a child is a severely stressful event that can have long-term disruptive effects on the family system. The family's ability to cope depends on family life patterns and on family structure, as well as on their social relations and use of community resources (Gary 1992; Reidy, Thibaudeau & Beauger 1995). The structure of the family may be composed of subgroups, such as the parenting subsystem, which provide nurturing, socialization and financial and social support of the child (Munson 1978). The child with AIDS often comes from a single-parent family, headed by a mother who is herself infected, her partner having abandoned her or having become incapacitated or died from AIDS himself. A second important subsystem in the family is the subgroup, such as the mother and daughter, which functions as a unit, sharing tasks and emotional support. This dyad is important in the family interaction with the child with terminal AIDS. It is often the grandmother who becomes a replacement natural caregiver and at times, primary nurturer.

A third important subgroup within the family is the sibling subsystem. A family that has one child dying of AIDS may well have other children who are healthy or who are also infected. The siblings of the terminally ill children live with illness, sorrow and death (Bluebond-Lagner 1989). They may experience change of roles and status and often have difficulty in obtaining the nurturing and attention they need as the infected child becomes sicker. They may see themselves as less favoured, even rejected. They may feel confused about their sibling's condition, their parents' emotions, who they are and what they should do. They are often unable to maintain their relationship with their sick sibling, particularly as the illness progresses and periods of hospitalization increase. They often face the death of the sibling with great ambivalence, particularly if they themselves are infected. They experience a variety of feelings including responsibility for the death of the sibling, resentment that the parents spent so much time with them, anger at the parents who let them die and fear that they themselves will be the next to die.

Dubik-Unruh (1989) has written of these children in the terminal phase of AIDS as being the children of chaos: dying children of dying families. By 'dying families', she means that not only have these families experienced multiple deaths, but also that they are in the process of dissolution from illness, hospitalization, abandonment, addiction, sibling separation, court removal of children, family breakup, homelessness and incarceration. The natural caregiver, that is, the mother, grandmother, foster parent or other surrogate nurturer of the child dying from AIDS, must envision the child's death in a social context tainted by social rejection. The social retreat enforced by such a situation renders the relation between caregiver and the sick person less and less satisfying. Consequently, there is a danger of premature disengagement and even abandonment by families. The stress of exigencies and the demands of the caregiving role are multiplied by the perceptions of burden in caregiving. Caregiving can provoke conflict in other roles and disrupt other areas of life (i.e. financial, occupational and social) which in turn become further sources of stress. In addition, the members of such families become incapable of giving the care and support needed as they suffer a gradual depletion of their physical, emotional and financial resources (Carmack 1992; Perreault and Savard 1992).

Natural caregivers of the child in the terminal phase of AIDS have lost most things that would help them face the mourning awaiting them. Implicated in an affective relationship with their child, which will culminate in death, they suffer from isolation, disorganization, stress, burnout and possibly mechanisms of adaptation which are inefficient or inadequate. In this emotional context, they have little chance of coming to terms with the loss of their child. Regardless of their feeling of preparedness, the death of a child provokes an intensive and difficult to resolve grief in the infected parent. Such parents frequently express suicidal ideation and the feeling that they have nothing to live for, they long to join their child in death (Anderson and Emery 1990; Weiner and Septimus 1991; Gary 1992).

The imminence of the death of her child also engenders a high level of stress in the HIV-infected mother who is also a caregiver, as it provokes the spectre of her own death and uncertainty about the future (Pearlin, Semple and Turner 1988; Boland 1990; Kaplan 1990; Septimus 1990). On the one hand, infected mothers have been found to be more concerned with the care of their child after their deaths, than with their own deaths (Reidy, Taggart and Asselin 1991). On the other hand, mothers from very different cultures maintain the belief, against 'great odds', that the medical research community, will find a treatment, if not a cure, in time for their child (Reidy et al 1995).

Moreover, the anticipated grief of an HIV-positive mother which follows on the deterioration of the health of the child in the terminal phase of AIDS, bears the promise of being dysfunctional. Their relationship is complicated not only by the practical difficulties of an HIV-positive caregiver caring for themselves and for a child, but also by the emotional problem of revealing the illness to family and friends, by the stigma of AIDS and possibly by a socially alienated life-style (O'Donnell 1992). Further, such grief, the expectation of loss before it occurs, is rendered more erratic by the interplay of uncertainty and hope provoked by the evolution of the illness in both caregiver and child (Mercier and Reidy 1995).

SALIENT ISSUES FOR THE CAREGIVERS OF THE BEREAVED OR DYING CHILD

Health is the result of the simultaneous presence of well-being and the absence of illness and implies congruency between the subjective perceptions of the individual and their family and the objective evaluation of the health system. Professional caregivers, such as the case-management nurse or social worker, assure the function of mediation between the objective-medical and the subjective-individual approaches. In order to do so, these professional caregivers must see the child and their family first as individuals and second as patients/families who are part of the established health system. The sick child, their natural caregiver and their professional caregiver (who varies from one health situation to another) form an interactive triad that takes charge of the health of the infected child or cares for the same child in the terminal phase of AIDS. The global aim of improving the child's quality of life depends on the development of a climate of confidence between members of this triad (Reidy and Taggart 1993).

Bonding between the Young Child and the Sick Mother

The mutual aim of bonding is attained between mother, perhaps sick herself, or surrogate caregiver and the infected infant by proximity and pleasurable interaction. The sick mother who tires easily can be encouraged to lie down with the child at nap or bedtime. She can be helped to devise ways in which they can enjoy themselves. Cuddling, massage, water play and tactile art are among the many interactive activities which are 'fun' for both. The parent or other natural caregiver can give physical care themselves if they are able, or participate in care, if they are not (i.e. holding the child when medication is given). During treatments, they should interact with the child rather than paying attention to the professional caregiver or to the treatment.

Communicating with the Bereaved or Dying Child

When is it right to tell the child that they are infected with HIV or dying from AIDS? or that family members are infected or have already died from the infection? What are the grounds for telling or not telling the child? Do the possible gains in long-term intimacy and psychological adjustment of disclosure, balance the increased anxiety that comes from knowing of a life-threatening illness? Are the health professionals' ethical and therapeutic responsibilities to the child in conflict with their responsibilities to the parents? While health professionals caring for the child with AIDS tend to favour disclosure and openness in communication, parents often fear disclosure and the ensuing discussion with their child. Conflictual or adversarial tendencies tend to confuse the issue and the child, whereas a three-way (child, parent and health professional) participation in a dialogue, helps all parties change and move the discussion from disclosure point to disclosure process (Lipson 1993).

The child's stage of development and preferred modality of communication is crucial during such discussions. As the child matures, the visual, the auditory and the kinetic become more interactive but, at the time of the stress of a great loss, what they see, what they hear, or what they feel, may assume the greater importance. When the best way to pass emotional or cognitive messages is unclear, multiple modes of communication, such as holding, talking, story-telling, using books or familiar objects are important.

Most literature on death and bereavement suggests openness of communication and some even rapid and direct confrontation of the finality of loss. However, confrontation should be adopted with caution and only under certain circumstances. Children and adolescents move with maturity toward the resolution of their losses. Forcing children to confront death or a terminal illness, particularly children with multiple losses associated with AIDS, could threaten their psychological integrity.

Surrogate and Foster Care

The child who has already lost one or both parents to AIDS bears the best chance to flourish if there is another nurturing person who will love and care for them. Knowing and feeling that someone will care for them will begin to alleviate the fundamental terror of being abandoned. If the child already knows and trusts the replacement caregiver, such as the remaining parent or a grandparent, or can come to know and accept the nurturing of a foster parent, and is allowed to express their grief, they have the possibility of coming to terms with their loss.

With the younger toddler or infant, the replacement nurturer can begin by fitting into the child's routine, within a familiar setting; the young child can be brought to experience a new setting through simple explanations, pictures, stories, books and temporary visits. Questions can be answered as clearly and honestly as possible and children of all ages can spend time with or actually visit their new homes on a regular basis.

Fortunately, the practice of keeping many of these infected infants in hospitals for extended periods of time has almost disappeared. Foster parents or long-term surrogate caregivers are being recruited through established child-service agencies, and group homes have been established by both volunteers and official organizations in both North America and Europe. These foster parents are usually required to have an understanding of AIDS, to have the time available, to be in good health, to have the space, to have no children under 10 and to have no serious interfering family or psychiatric problems (Mock 1989; Rendon et al 1991; Taylor-Brown 1991).

Issues surrounding the placement and acceptance of HIV-positive children include the risk of foster parents becoming caught up in a cycle of multiple losses, grief, mourning and eventually burnout. There is the fear of spread of infection and the powerful emotional and social implications of the social stigma associated with AIDS. Further, not only do the foster parents bear the burden of caring for a chronically ill child, with all the attending care and treatment requirements, but also these children may demonstrate developmental delay, behavioural regression, and in the case of older children, behavioural and psychological problems.

Anticipatory Grief of the Natural Caregivers of the Child in the Terminal Phase of AIDS

As the child known to be infected becomes symptomatic, the grieving process begins when the mourner accepts the reality of the loss through observation of the physical decline. The anticipation of grief is part of the normal grieving process, which is triggered through the anticipation of death and its consequences. Gradual withdrawal, divesting of roles and ties, completion of joint tasks, expression of emotions or resolution of conflicts, are often used by families in their relations with the person who is terminally ill. This process is positive and qualitatively different from premature detachment, which can leave the dying person abandoned emotionally or physically, and the mourner guilty with their grief unresolved (Rando 1988). It can, in the context of healthy mourning, improve the mourner's capacity to adapt and help in the relation between the sick person and those close to him. Supporting the dying child can make the distress of the grief process less acute (Régnier 1991).

Inspired by the work of Bowlby (1981), Worden (1991) has proposed a model of anticipated grief and grief counselling, in the context of group interaction, which has been applied effectively with the natural caregivers of men in the terminal phase of AIDS (Fontaine and Reidy 1995). The social support, provided through the group, becomes a therapeutic intervention between the health professional and the mourners as well as between mourners themselves. This social support becomes complementary to the repertoire of relationships from which the mourner is likely to procure diverse forms of aid. The process of anticipated grief represents a personal adaptive response to stress and can serve as a shield against the burdens of caregiving in the terminal phase of AIDS.

The denial of the loss, the sense of unreality and the suffering of the caregivers of the child dying from AIDS, are also likely to respond to the process of anticipated grief. Following the death of the child, it will allow the caregivers to adjust more readily to the environment and life situation where the loved child is absent rather than to respond by flight in realizing the immensity of their loss. They will be better prepared, eventually, to withdraw emotional energy from dealing with the loss of the child and to redirect this energy toward different relations and activities. This is of particular importance if the caregiver himself or herself, or other members of the family, is infected, because they will require that time and energy be devoted towards their health and well-being.

THE FUTURE: INTERVENTION AND CONCEPTUAL ISSUES

Family Competencies

A wide range of interventions need to be developed to respond to the needs of the bereaved and the dying child. These interventions must take into account the evolution of the disease process, the stages of development and the needs and abilities of the caregivers, in order to improve the quality of all their lives. The response of health professionals to the family, or most importantly to that family member (or surrogate) who plays the role of primary nurturer and caregiver, is a deciding factor in the role played by the family during the terminal phase of the child's illness. Families of HIV-infected children, because of social alienation, high-risk life-styles or just because of the stigma of infection, may lose even recognition that they love and care about their children. Moreover, the primary nurturers who assume the burden of caregiving, in extended families, are often refused the status of family. These caregivers may be denied the right to be partners in the decisions which affect the child's care in their terminal illness and in the manner of dying (National Pediatric HIV Resource Center 1992).

We need to be concerned with issues such as advocacy, empowerment, actualization and self-efficacy, and changes in values and attitudes, even if, at times, it places us, the professional caregivers, in a functional limbo between the family of the child infected with HIV and the established medical/health system (Reidy 1995).

The role of advocate entails helping the family affected with HIV to clarify their values and come to appropriate decisions based on these values, as well as helping them to find the means to manage the difficult situations in which they find themselves. It means helping them understand how the health and welfare system works and how to use it appropriately. Advocacy does not remove the responsibility from the family to act; rather its aim is to promote family autonomy in health matters and to facilitate the learning of new behaviours which are conducive to independence.

Empowerment is a social process that is crucial to families affected with HIV, who have been disempowered by poverty, stigma and alienation.

It is concerned with control, mastery, rights and authority. It strengthens the mediating structures between individuals and societies and even encourages the changing of the structures rather than just integration into existing structures. Through social participation and negotiation, it counters social isolation, extends the family's social network, increases their control in social interactions (including interaction with health professionals) and expands their access to new resources. As part of this process, the child and the natural caregiver can be encouraged to become involved in new social situations such as playgroups, self-help groups, social and recreative groups, political action groups, etc.

Caregivers and nurturers of the child dying of AIDS will only be as competent as they believe themselves to be. Perception of self-efficacy (expectations of success) determines, in great part, whether or not a person will engage in a given behaviour. Learned through personal or vicarious experience, verbal persuasion and physical feedback, self-efficacy is directly related to competency. Improving the caregivers' competencies and their perception of their ability to succeed will improve the quality of care given to the child and ease the burden felt by the caregiver (Bandura 1977).

Care for the Dying Child

Relaxation and mild exercise can improve the welfare of both the caregiver and the child, particularly if these activities become part of their lives early in the infection. However, while the effect of 'alternate' therapies has rarely been described for children in the terminal phase of AIDS, their utility in symptom relief and even their relation to immunostatus have been reported for infected adults (Solomon et al 1987; Carr 1991; Evans 1991; Lang 1993). While visualization, massage, music and meditation have demonstrated their effectiveness as complementary therapies to medical treatment regimens, they are often slow to be mastered or accepted in acute care settings.

No instruments seem, as yet, to have been developed and published to evaluate pain, and few specific drug protocols have been devised specifically in response to pain in the child with terminal AIDS. Most hospital clinicians seem to rely on habitual paediatric pain control medications or to turn for consultation in pain management to paediatric oncological teams. Hospice caregivers, however, long cognizant of the importance of symptom management for children dying of other chronic diseases, such as cancer or leukaemia, have begun to apply these approaches to children dying of AIDS. Moreover, home-care nurses, and the AIDS-care multidisciplinary teams with whom they work, have given priority to helping parents and surrogate natural caregivers manage symptoms of children in the terminal phase who remain at home (Boland and Klug 1986; Daily 1991; Boland and Conviser 1992).

Conceptual and Psychometric Issues: Concept of Death and Dying

There would seem to be a need to broaden both the psychometric and theoretical purview of work in the domain related to death and the child infected with HIV. The development of qualitative approaches (i.e. pheno-menographic methodology) and standardized validated instruments (i.e. the *Death Concept Questionnaire*, Smilansky (1981), and the *Derry Death Scale*, Derry (1979)), will allow research on children and death, in the future, to evolve from the traditional structured interview and projective techniques (Prichard and Epting 1991–1992). Methodological developments such as these equip us better to answer the questions we need to ask.

The current body of research in the domain of children and death has been focused, in great part, on concept formation and bereavement in healthy children. We also have some knowledge of the thoughts and experiences of children with other chronic illnesses such as leukaemia, cancer or cystic fibrosis, but little of the social world of children who are seriously ill and dying of AIDS. The long-term survivors of childhood HIV infection have had years of interaction with their peers in waiting rooms and hospital units. These children will, to some extent, develop and maintain peer relations based on health condition rather than on friendship and support. Relationships with healthy peers are difficult to maintain with frequent illnesses and possible disruption in pattern of growth and development. Family relationships and structures are also disrupted by the impact of the chronic and fatal nature of the HIV disease process. Moreover, understanding the social world of children with AIDS is particularly important because the disease itself is symbolically charged, the children have contracted it from a stigmatized population, the parents of these children are also likely to be dead or dying and these children come, in great part, from poor, alienated or marginal ethnic groups (Bluebond-Lagner 1992).

Further, while death anxiety or threat is well represented in the adult literature, relatively few such studies have been reported about children. At what point in the evolution of an illness, such as AIDS, do children, as compared with healthy children, develop death threat? What role do the particular social factors of stigma and isolation play in death anxieties? Is there a particular relationship between the death anxieties of the HIV-infected parent and child? We also need to comprehend the conceptualization of the concept of death and dying, of children infected with HIV within the interactive context of their cognitive development, their social world and the evolution of the disease process. If we are to respond to them as they confront death, their own or perhaps those close to them, it is important to understand death as the child understands it.

REFERENCES

Abrams EJ & Nicholas SW (1990) Pediatric HIV infection *Pediatr Ann* **19**: 482–7

American Academy of Pediatrics – Task Force on Pediatrics (1989) Infants and children with Acquired Immunodeficiency Syndrome: placement in adoption and foster care *Pediatrics* **83**: 609–12

Anderson GR & Emery J (1990) Present and future challenges in caring for children with HIV and their families. In R Anderson (ed) *Courage to Care* Washington: Child Welfare League of America pp 305–19

Anthony S (1972) *The Discovery of Death in Childhood and After* New York: Basic Books

Bacqué MF (1992) *Le Deuil à Vivre* Paris: Editions Odile Jacob

Bandura A (1977) *Social Learning Theory* Englewood Cliffs, NJ: Prentice Hall

Binger CM, Ablin AR, Feuerstein RC et al (1969) Childhood leukemia: emotional impact on patient and family *N Engl J Med* **208**: 414–18

Bluebond-Lagner M (1977) Meanings of death to children. In H Fiefel (ed) *New Meanings of Death* New York: McGraw-Hill pp 47–66

Bluebond-Lagner M (1989) Worlds of dying children and their well siblings *Death Stud* **13**: 1–16

Bluebond-Lagner M (1992) Children and death: direction for the 90s *Loss Grief Care* **6**: 61–72

Boland MG (1990) Supporting families caring for children with HIV infection. In R Anderson (ed) *Courage to Care* Washington: Child Welfare League of America pp 65–76

Boland MG & Klug RM (1986) AIDS: the implications for home care *Am J Mat Child* **11**: 404–11

Boland MG & Conviser R (1992) Nursing care of the child. In JH Flaskerud & PJ Ungvarski (eds) *HIV/AIDS: A Guide to Nursing Care* (2nd edn) Philadelphia: WB Saunders pp 199–238

Bourdeau M (1986) Elaboration et verification d'un instrument d'évaluation de la relation entre la mère et le nouveau-né *Rapport de maîtrise* Faculté des Sciences Infirmières, Université de Montréal (unpublished)

Bourdeau M & Taggart ME (1995) L'attachement maternel et l'infection par le VIH. In M Reidy & ME Taggart (eds) *VIH/SIDA: Une Approche Heuristique. Réflexions et Stratégies pour les Professionnels de la Santé* Montréal: Gaëtan Morin Editeur in press

Bowlby J (1971a) *Attachment and Loss, Vol. I: Attachment* Harmondsworth: Penguin

Bowlby J (1971b) *Attachment and Loss, Vol. II: Separation* Harmondsworth: Penguin

Bowlby J (1981) *Attachment and Loss, Vol. III: Loss, sadness and depression* Harmondsworth: Penguin

Boyd-Franklin N & Aleman J (1990) Black, inner-city families and multigenerational issues: the impact of AIDS *Psychology* **40**(3): 14–17

Carmack BJ (1992) Balancing engagement/detachment in AIDS-related multiple losses *Image: J Nurs Schol* **24**: 9–14

Carr G (1991) Nursing beliefs and pain management *Nurs Stand* **5**(40 Suppl): 54–5

Combs AW, Richards AC & Richards F (1976) *Perceptual Psychology: A Humanistic Approach to the Study of Persons* New York: Harper and Row

Corr CA (1992) A task-based approach to coping with dying *Omega* **24**: 81–94

Daily AA (1991) Terminal care for the child with AIDS. In PA Pizzo & CM Wilfred (eds) *Pediatric AIDS* Baltimore: Williams and Wilkins pp 619–29

Derry SM (1979) *An Empirical Investigation of Death in Children* Doctoral Thesis, Ottawa University, Canada

Dickinson GE (1992) First childhood death experiences *Omega* **25**: 169–82

Dubik-Unruh S (1989) Children of chaos: planning for the emotional survival of dying children of dying families *J Palliat Care* **5**(2): 10–15

Dyregrov A (1991) *Grief in Children: A Handbook for Adults* London: Jessica Kingsley

Evans G (1991) A wider perspective in symptom relief *Nurs Stand* **6**(1 Suppl) 50–1

Fassler D, McQueen K, Duncan P & Copeland L (1990) Children's perceptions of AIDS *J Am Acad Child Adolesc Psychiatry* **29**: 259–62

Fontaine G & Reidy M (1995) L'anticipation du deuil chez les soignants naturels de sidéens en phase invalidante: une analyse et un programme d'intervention. In M Reidy & ME Taggart (eds) *VIH/SIDA: Une Approche Heuristique. Réflexions et Stratégies pour les Professionnels de la Santé* Montréal: Gaëtan Morin Editeur in press

Furman E (1974) *A Child's Parent Dies: Studies in Childhood Bereavement* New Haven, CT: Yale University Press

Furman E (1984) Children's pattern of mourning the death of a loved one. In H Wass & C Corr (eds) *Childhood and Death* Washington: Hemisphere pp 185–204

Gary GA (1992) Facing terminal illness in children with AIDS *Home Healthcare Nurse* **10**(2): 40–3

Glebatis DM, Novick LF & Stacy BA (1991) VIII. Hospitalization of HIV-seropositive newborns with AIDS-related diseases within the first year of life *Am J Pub Health* **81**(Suppl): 46–9

Green J & Sherr L (1989) Dying, bereavement and loss. In J Green (ed) *Counselling in AIDS* London: Blackwell Scientific pp 207–23

Guy T (1993) Exploratory study of elementary aged children's conceptions of death through the use of story *Death Stud* **17**: 27–54

Halprin EN (1993) Denial in children whose parents died of AIDS *Child Psychiatry Hum Dev* **23**(4): 249–57

Hauger SB & Powell KR (1990) Infectious complications in children with HIV infection *Pediatr Ann* **19**: 421–36

Hostler SL (1978) The development of the child's concept of death. In OJZ Sahler (ed) *The Child and Death* St Louis: CV Mosby pp 1–25

Hug-Hellmuth VH (1965) The child's concept of death *Psychoanal Q* **34**: 499–516

Jewett CL (1982) *Helping Children Cope With Loss* Harvard, MA: Harvard Common Press

Kane B (1979) Children's concepts of death *J Genet Psychol* **134**: 141–53

Kaplan M (1990) Psychosocial issues of children and families with HIV/AIDS *Occup Ther Child Care* **7**: 139–42

Kastenbaum E (1977) Death and development through the life-span. In H Feifel (ed) *New Meanings of Death* New York: McGraw-Hill pp 17–45

Kubler-Ross E (1969) *On Death and Dying* New York: Macmillan

Kubler-Ross E (1983) *On Children and Death* New York: Macmillan

Lang C (1993) Using relaxation and exercise as part of the care of people living with HIV/AIDS *Physiotherapy* **79**: 379–84

Levine C & Dubler NN (1990) Uncertain risks and bitter realities: the reproductive choices of HIV-infected women *Millbank Q* **68**: 321–51

Lipson M (1993) What do you say to a child with AIDS? *Hastings Center Rep* **23**(2): 6–12

Lonetto R (1980) *Children's Concepts of Death* New York: Springer

McClain KL & Rosenblett H (1990) Pediatric HIV infection and AIDS: clinical expression of malignancy *Semin Pediatr Infect Dis* **1**: 124–9

McCown DE (1988) When children face death in a family *J Pediatr Health Care* **2**: 14–19

McElreath LH & Roberts MC (1991) Perceptions of acquired immune deficiency syndrome by children and their parents *J Pediatr Psychol* **17**: 477–90

Maurer A (1966) Maturation of the concept of death *J Med Psychol* **39**: 35–42

Meintz SL & Lynch RD (1989) The human right of bonding for warehoused AIDS babies *Family Community Health* **12**(2): 60–4

Melvin D & Sherr L (1993) The child in the family – responding to AIDS and HIV *AIDS Care* **5**: 35–42

Mercier L & Reidy M (1995) Incertitude et espoir auprès des personnes vivant avec le VIH. In M Reidy & ME Taggart (eds) *VIH/SIDA: une Approche Heuristique. Réflexions et Stratégies pour les Professionnels de la Santé* Montréal: Gaëtan Morin Editeur in press

Mock J (1989) Pediatric HIV infection. In J Green (ed) *Counselling in AIDS* London: Blackwell Scientific pp 157–66

Mock J, Giaquinto C, Derossi A et al (1987) Infants born to mothers seropositive for Human Immunodeficiency Virus: preliminary findings from a multicentre European study *Lancet* i: 1164–8

Monbourquette J (1992) *Comment pardonner?* Ottawa: Novalis

Munson SW (1978) Family structure and the family's general adaptation to loss: helping families deal with the death of a child. In OJZ Sahler (ed) *The Child and Death* St Louis: CV Mosby pp 29–42

Murphy P & Perry K (1988) Hidden grievers *Death Stud* **12**: 451–62

Nagy M (1948) The child's theories concerning death *J Genet Psychol* **73**: 3–27

National Pediatric HIV Resource Center – Task Force on Pediatric AIDS (1992) *Getting A Head Start on HIV: A Resource Manual for Enhancing Services to HIV Affected Children in Head Start* Newark, NJ: National Pediatric HIV Resource Center

O'Donnell MC (1992) Loss, grief, and growth. In MR Seligson & KE Peterson (eds) *AIDS, Prevention and Treatment: Hope, Humor and Healing* New York: Hemisphere

Parkes CM (1979) *Bereavement. Studies of Grief in Adult Life* New York: International Universities Press

Parry JK & Thornwall J (1992) Death of a father *Death Stud* **16**: 173–81

Pearlin LI, Semple S & Turner H (1988) Stress of AIDS caregivers: a preliminary overview of issues *Death Stud* **12**: 501–17

Penson J (1990) *Bereavement. Studies of Grief in Adult Life* London: Harper and Row

Perreault M & Savard N (1992) Le vécu et l'implication d'aidants naturels de personnes vivants avec le VIH *Santé Ment Québec* **17**: 111–30

Piaget J (1973) *The Child and Reality – Problems of Genetic Psychology* New York: Grossman

Pizzo PA & Wilfert CM (1991) *Pediatric AIDS: The Challenge of HIV Infection In Infants, Children and Adolescents* Baltimore: Williams and Wilkins

Prichard S & Epting F (1991–1992) Children and death *Omega* **24**: 271–88

Rando T (1984) *Grief, Dying and Death: Clinical Interventions for Caregivers* Champaign: Research Press

Rando T (1988) *Grieving. How to Go on Living When Someone You Love Dies* Lexington: Lexington Books

Régnier R (1991) *La Perte d'un Être Cher. Le Travail de Deuil* Montréal: Les Editions Québécor

Reidy M (1995) Proposition d'un modèle infirmier en santé communautaire visant l'amélioration des compétences de familles à charge d'enfants atteints par le VIH. In M Reidy & ME Taggart (eds) *VIH/SIDA: Une Approche Heuristique. Réflexions et Stratégies pour les Professionnels de la Santé* Montréal: Gaëtan Morin Editeur in press

Reidy M & Taggart ME (1993) Un modèle de soins infirmiers auprès de familles d'enfants infectés par le VIH *Bull Prise Charge* 3(1): 3

Reidy M, Taggart ME & Asselin L (1991) Psychosocial needs expressed by the natural caregivers of HIV infected children *AIDS Care* 3: 345–53

Reidy M, Thibaudeau MF & Beauger M (1995) Elaboration et validation de l'échelle d'Evaluation du Fonctionnement de la Famille en matière de santé (EFF). In M Reidy & ME Taggart (eds) *VIH/SIDA: Une Approche Heuristique. Réflexions et Stratégies pour les Professionnels de la Santé* Montréal: Gaëtan Morin Editeur in press

Reidy M, Taggart ME, Deslongchamps A et al (1995) Résultats de l'application du modèle auprès de deux familles d'ethnie différente. In M Reidy & ME Taggart (eds) *VIH/SIDA: Une Approche Heuristique. Réflexions et Stratégies pour les Professionnels de la Santé* Montréal: Gaëtan Morin Editeur in press

Rendon M, Gurdin P, Bassi J & Weston M (1991) Foster care for children with AIDS: a psychosocial perspective *Child Psychiatry Hum Dev* 19: 256–69

Rogers CR (1991) A theory of therapy, personality and interpersonal relationship as developed in the client centered framework. In S Koch (ed) *Psychology: A Study of Science* (Vol 3) New York: McGraw-Hill pp 184–256

Schvaneveldt JD, Lindauer SLK & Young MH (1990) Children's understanding of AIDS: a developmental viewpoint *Family Rel* 39: 330–5

Septimus A (1990) Caring for HIV-infected children and their families: psychosocial ramification. In *Courage to Care* Washington: Child Welfare League of America pp 99–106

Sherr L (1991) *HIV and AIDS in Mothers and Babies* London: Blackwell Scientific

Sigelman C, Maddock A, Epstein J & Carpenter W (1993) Age difference in understanding of disease causality: AIDS, colds and cancer *Child Dev* 64: 272–84

Sly DF, Eberstein IW, Quadagno D & Kistner KA (1992) Young children's awareness, knowledge and beliefs about AIDS: observation from a pretest. *AIDS Educ Prev* 4: 227–9

Smilannky SN (1981) *Manual for Questionnaire of the Development of Death Conceptualization.* Unpublished manuscript, University of Tel Aviv

Solomon GR, Temoshok L, O'Leary A & Zich J (1987) An intensive psychoimmunologic study of long-surviving persons with AIDS *Ann N Y Acad Sci* 496: 647–55

Spinetta JJ & Malony LJ (1975) Death anxiety in the outpatient leukemic child *Pediatrics* 56: 1034–7

Stroebe M (1992–1993) Coping with bereavement: a review of the grief work hypothesis *Omega* 26: 19–42

Taylor-Brown S (1991) The impact of AIDS on foster care: a family centered approach to services in the United States *Child Welfare* 70: 193–209

Viney LL, Henry RM, Walker BM & Crooks L (1992) The psychosocial impact of multiple deaths from AIDS *Omega* 24: 151–63

Waechter EH (1971) Children's awareness of fatal illness *Am J Nurs* 71(6): 1168–72

Waechter EH (1984) Dying children: patterns of coping. In H Wass & C Corr (eds) *Childhood and Death* Washington: Hemisphere pp 51–68

Waechter EH, Chittenden M, Mikkelsen C & Holaday B (1986) Concomitants of death imagery in stories told by chronically ill children undergoing intrusive procedures: a comparison of four diagnostic groups *J Pediatr Nurs* 1: 2–11

Walsh ME & Bibace R (1991) Children's conceptions of AIDS: a developmental analysis *J Pediatr Psychol* **16**: 273–85

Wass H (1984) Concept of death: a developmental perspective. In H Wass & C Corr (eds) *Childhood and Death* Washington: Hemisphere pp 3–21

Wass H & Scott M (1978) Middle schools students' concepts and concerns *Mid School J* **9**: 10–12

Wass H & Cason L (1984) Fears and anxieties about death. In H Wass & C Corr (eds) *Childhood and Death* Washington: Hemisphere pp 25–45

Weiner L & Septimus A (1991) Psychosocial consideration and support for the child and the family. In PA Pizzo & CM Wilfert (eds) *Pediatric AIDS: The Challenge of HIV Infection in Infants, Children and Adolescents* Baltimore: Williams and Wilkins pp 576–94

Wiznia AA & Nicholas SW (1990) Organ system involvement in HIV-infected children *Pediatr Ann* **19**: 475–81

Worden JW (1991) *Grief Counseling and Grief Therapy* New York: Springer

Index

Wiley Titles of Related Interest

CANCER AND EMOTION
A Practical Guide to Psycho-oncology
2nd Edition
Jennifer Barraclough
Helps professionals working with cancer patients understand the emotional aspects of cancer, and the specialised interventions that are available.

0-471-93721-5   198pp   paper 1994

SURVIVING GRIEF AND LEARNING TO LIVE AGAIN
Catherine M. Sanders
Defines and explains the five distinct phases—shock, awareness of loss, conservation and the need to withdraw, healing, and renewal—and offers compassionate guidance for working through each stage of the mourning process.

0-471-53471-4   238pp   paper 1992

GRIEF
The Mourning After—Dealing with Adult Bereavement
Catherine M. Sanders
Focuses on practical applications for caregiving to those suffering from grief, to help health professionals gain a better understanding of the process of bereavement.

0-471-62728-3   272pp   cloth 1989

PSYCHO-ONCOLOGY
Journal of the Psychological, Social and Behavioral Dimensions of Cancer
Editors: Jimmie Holland *and* Maggie Watson
Covers topics of research, clinical and theoretical interest, relating to the psycho-social aspects of cancer and AIDS-related tumors.

ISSN: 1057–9249

AIDS CARE AT HOME
A Guide for Caregivers, Loved Ones and People with AIDS
Judith Greif *and* Beth Ann Golden
Takes a positive approach to AIDS care for both the patient and carer and details everything from nutrition and medicine to the latest drugs and therapies and the emotional problems that surround this devastating disease.

0-471-58468-1   1994   380pp   paper